ASKLEPIOS
THEMATIC LIBRARY

FIRST AID

Paramount Books (Pvt.) Ltd.

Karachi | Lahore | Islamabad | Sukkur | Faisalabad | Peshawar | Abbottabad

ASKLEPIOS
THEMATIC LIBRARY

FIRST AID

Paramount Books (Pvt.) Ltd.

Karachi | Lahore | Islamabad | Sukkur | Faisalabad | Peshawar | Abbottabad

© Asklepios Medical Atlas

Asklepios Thematic Library First Aids 2016
by
Jordi Vigue

This edition has been published in arrangement with Asklepios Medical Atlas Barcelona, Spain

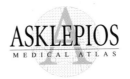

ASKLEPIOS
MEDICAL ATLAS

Paramount Books (Pvt.) Ltd.

152/O, Block-2, P.E.C.H.S., Karachi-75400. Tel: 34310030
Fax: 34553772, E-mail: info@paramountbooks.com.pk
Website: www.paramountbooks.com.pk

ISBN: 978-969-637-156-4

Printed in Pakistan

ASKLEPIOS MEDICAL ATLAS
SCIENTIFIC ADVISORS

General coordinator

Ricard Ramos Izquierdo
Specialist in Thoracic Surgery, Hospital Universitari de Bellvitge, l'Hospitalet de Llobregat, Barcelona. Associated Professor in Human Anatomy and Embriology, Universitat de Barcelona.

Scientific advisors and collaborators

Andrés Alvarado Segovia
Sports Medicine Specialist,
Bodytech, Bogotá.

Josep M. de Anta Vinyals
Associate Professor in Anatomy
and Human Embriology,
Campus de Ciències de la Salut
de Bellvitge,
Universitat de Barcelona.

Montse Arnán Sangermán
Specialist in Hematology,
Servei d'Hematologia Clínica,
Hospital Duran i Reynals,
Institut Català d'Oncologia,
l'Hospitalet de Llobregat, Barcelona.

Samantha Aso González
Specialist in Pneumology,
Servei de Neumologia,
Hospital Universitari de Bellvitge,
l'Hospitalet de Llobregat, Barcelona.

Llorenç Balagueró i Lladó
Former Chief of the Gynecology Unit
Hospital Universitari de Bellvitge,
l'Hospitalet de Llobregat, Barcelona.
Tenured Professor in Obstetrics
and Gynecology,
Facultat de Medicina,
Universitat de Barcelona.

Carme Baliellas i Comellas
Specialist of the Digestive Department,
Hospital Universitari de Bellvitge,
l'Hospitalet de Llobregat, Barcelona.

Cristina Berdié i Rabanaque
Specialist in Obstetrics and Gynecology,
Hospital General de l'Hospitalet de Llobregat,
Barcelona.

Jordi Bermúdez i Mas
Professor in Biophysics,
Departament de Ciències Fisiològiques II.
Universitat de Barcelona.

Marc Blasi i Brugué
Associate Professor in Human Anatomy,
Grau d'Infermeria, Laboratori
d'Anatomia Ecogràfica,
Facultat de Medicina
(Campus de Bellvitge),
Universitat de Barcelona.

Enric Buendia i Gràcia
Former Chief of the Immunology
Department,
Hospital Universitari de Bellvitge,
l'Hospitalet de Llobregat, Barcelona.

Mònica Buxeda i Rodríguez
Licenciate in Medicine,
Universitat de Barcelona.
Collaborator and Research Worker
in Human Anatomy,
Unitat d'Anatomia Humana,
Facultat de Medicina,
Hospital Universitari de Bellvitge,
l'Hospitalet de Llobregat, Barcelona.

Xavier Cabo Cabo
Specialist in Orthopaedic Surgery
and Traumatology,
Chief of the Septics Functional
Department,
Hospital Universitari de Bellvitge,
l'Hospitalet de Llobregat, Barcelona.
Associate Professor in Orthopaedic
Surgery and Traumatology,
Universitat de Barcelona.

Josep M. Caminal i Mitjana
Specialist in Ophthalmology,
Hospital Universitari de Bellvitge,
l'Hospitalet de Llobregat, Barcelona.
Associate Professor in Ophthalmology,
Universitat de Barcelona.

Anna Carrera Burgaya
Tenured Professor in Human Anatomy
and Embriology,
Departament de Ciències Mèdiques.
Universitat de Girona.

Maria Lluïsa Catasús i Clavé
Specialist in Rehabilitation,
Hospital Universitari de Bellvitge,
l'Hospitalet de Llobregat, Barcelona.

Manuel Chiva Royo
Tenured Professor in Physiology,
Departament de Fisiología,
Universitat de Barcelona.

Marta Andrea Díaz Ferrer
Resident Physician in Pneumology,
Servei de Neumologia,
Hospital Universitari de Bellvitge,
l'Hospitalet de Llobregat, Barcelona.

Josep Ramon Farreres i Riera
Specialist in Dermatology,
Hospital Universitari de Bellvitge,
l'Hospitalet de Llobregat, Barcelona.

Albert Francès i Comalat
Specialist in Urology,
Hospital del Mar, Barcelona.
Associate Professor in Urology,
Universitat Autònoma de Barcelona.
Universitat Pompeu Fabra,
Barcelona.

Eladio Franco Miranda
Former Chief of Urology Department,
Hospital Universitari de Bellvitge,
l'Hospitalet de Llobregat, Barcelona.
Associate Professor in Urology,
Universitat de Barcelona.

Xavier Fulladosa i Oliveras
Specialist in Nephrology,
Hospital Universitari de Bellvitge,
l'Hospitalet de Llobregat, Barcelona.

José Manual Gómez Sáez
Chief of the Endocrinology
and Nutrition Department,
Hospital Universitari de Bellvitge,
l'Hospitalet de Llobregat, Barcelona.
Associate Professor in Endocrinology,
Universitat de Barcelona.

Jordi Guardiola i Capó
Chief of the Gastro-intestinal Department,
Hospital Universitari de Bellvitge,
l'Hospitalet de Llobregat,
Barcelona.

José Antonio Hernández Hermoso
Chief of the Orthopaedic Surgery
and Traumatology Department,
Hospital Germans Trias i Pujol,
Badalona, Barcelona.

Francisco Jara Sureda
Specialist in Cardiology.
Hospital Universitari de Bellvitge,
l'Hospitalet de Llobregat, Barcelona.

Serge Jaumà Classen
Specialist in Neurology.
Unitat de Trastorns del Moviment.
Hospital Universitari de Bellvitge.
Professor of Human Physiology.
Departament d'Infermeria
Fundamental i Medicoquirúrgica.
Campus de Bellvitge,
Universitat de Barcelona.

Casimiro Fco. Javierre Garcés
Specialist in Medicine of Sport,
Associate Professor,
Unitat de Fisiologia,
Departament de Ciències Fisiològiques II,
Universitat de Barcelona.

Xavier Juanola i Roura
Chief of the Rheumatology Department,
Hospital Universitari de Bellvitge,
l'Hospitalet de Llobregat, Barcelona.
Profesor de Reumatología,
Universitat de Barcelona.

Jerky Krupinski
Specialist in Neurology,
Hospital Mútua de Terrassa,
Terrassa, Barcelona.

Iván Macía Vidueira
Specilist in Thoracic Surgery,
Hospital Universitari de Bellvitge.
Associate Professor, Grau d'Infermeria,
Universitat de Barcelona.

Frederic Manresa i Presas
Chief of the Pneumology Department,
Hospital Universitari de Bellvitge,
Barcelona.
Tenured Professor in Pneumology,
Universitat de Barcelona.

M. Cristina Manzanares Céspedes
Tenured Professor in Human Anatomy
and Embriology,
Campus de Ciències de la Salut
de Bellvitge,
l'Hospitalet de Llobregat, Barcelona.

M. Isabel Miguel Pérez
Tenured Professor in Human Anatomy
and Embriology,
Campus de Ciències de la Salut
de Bellvitge,
l'Hospitalet de Llobregat, Barcelona.

Júlia Miró i Lladó
Specialist in Neurology,
Unitat d'Epilèpsies,
Hospital Universitari de Bellvitge,
l'Hospitalet de Llobregat, Barcelona.

Jaume Ordi i Majà
Specialist in Pathologic Anatomy,
Servei d'Anatomia Patològica,
Hospital Clínic de Barcelona, Barcelona.

Jaume Pahisa i Fàbregas
Specialist in Obstetrics and Gynecology,
Servei de Ginecología,
Hospital Clínic de Barcelona, Barcelona.

Raquel Pascual Cascón
Specialist in Pneumology,
Servei de Neumologia,
Hospital Universitari de Bellvitge,
l'Hospitalet de Llobregat, Barcelona.

Rosa M. Penín Mosquera
Specialist in Pathologic Anatomy,
Servei d'Anatomia Patològica,
Hospital Universitari de Bellvitge,
l'Hospitalet de Llobregat, Barcelona.

Joan Pericas i Bosch
Specialist in Pediatrics.

Elena Pina i Pascual
Specialist in Hematology,
Àrea de Trombosi i Hemostàsia,
Hospital Universitari de Bellvitge,
l'Hospitalet de Llobregat, Barcelona.

Marta del Pino Saladrigues
Specialist in Obstetrics and Gynecology,
Institut Clínic de Ginecologia,
Obstetrícia i Neonatologia (ICGON),
Hospital Clínic de Barcelona, Barcelona.

Jordi Prat i Ortells
Specialist in Pediatric Surgery,
Secció de Cirugía Neonatal,
Hospital de Sant Joan de Déu,
Barcelona.

Albert Prats i Galino
Professor of Human Pathologic Anatomy,
Universitat de Barcelona.

Manuel Ramos Izquierdo
DO Osteopathic and Sport
Physiotherapy,
Professor of Physiotherapeutic Grade.
Universitat Ramon Llull,
Institut Ramos Izquierdo,
Barcelona

Emilio Ramos Rubio
Chief of the General
and Gastro-intestinal Surgery,
Secció de Cirugía General i Digestiva,
Unitat de Trasplantament Hepàtic,
Hospital Universitari de Bellvitge, Barcelona.
Tenured Professor in Surgery,
Universitat de Barcelona.

Jordi Rancaño Ferreiro
Former Chief of the Angiology and Vascular
Surgery Department,
Hospital Universitari de Bellvitge,
l'Hospitalet de Llobregat, Barcelona.

Purificación Regueiro Espín
Specialist in Obstetrics and Gynecology,
Hospital General de l'Hospitalet de Llobregat,
Barcelona.

Xavier Rius i Moreno
Specialist in Orthopaedic Surgery
and Traumatology,
Hospital Universitari de Bellvitge,
l'Hospitalet de Llobregat, Barcelona.

Francisco Rivas Doyague
Specialist in Thoracic Surgery,
Hospital Universitari de Bellvitge,
l'Hospitalet de Llobregat, Barcelona.

Josep Rodríguez i Tolrà
Specialist in Urology,
Chief of the Andrology Department,
Erectile Dysfunction and Urethral
Pathology Department,
Hospital Universitari de Bellvitge,
l'Hospitalet de Llobregat, Barcelona.

Carla Rojas Bautista
Specialist in Obstetrics and Gynecology,
Zita West Assisted Fertility, Londres.

Montserrat Romera Baures
Specialist in Rheumatology,
Servei de Reumatologia
Hospital Universitari de Bellvitge,
l'Hospitalet de Llobregat, Barcelona.

Antonio Romera Villegas
Specialist in Angiology and Vascular Surgery,
Hospital Universitari de Bellvitge,
l'Hospitalet de Llobregat,
Barcelona.

Lucía Romero-Pinell
Specialist in Neurology,
Unitat d'Esclerosi Múltiple
Hospital Universitari de Bellvitge,
l'Hospitalet de Llobregat, Barcelona.

Antoni Rozadilla Sacanell
Specialist in Rheumatology,
Servei de Reumatologia
Hospital Universitari de Bellvitge,
l'Hospitalet de Llobregat, Barcelona.

Francisco Rubio Borrego
Chief of Neurology Department,
Hospital Universitari de Bellvitge,
l'Hospitalet de Llobregat, Barcelona.
Tenured Professor in Neurology,
Universitat de Barcelona.

Xavier Sabaté de la Cruz
Chief of the Cardiology Department,
Unitat d'Arrítmies,
Hospital Universitari de Bellvitge,
l'Hospitalet de Llobregat, Barcelona.

Margalida E Sastre Cuadrí
Specialist in Obstetrics
and Gynecology,
Hospital General de l'Hospitalet,
l'Hospitalet de Llobregat, Barcelona.

Ramon Segura i Cardona
Professor Emeritus of Physiology,
Universitat de Barcelona.

Octavi Servitje Bedate
Specialist in Dermatology,
Hospital Universitari de Bellvitge,
l'Hospitalet de Llobregat, Barcelona.
Associate Professor in Dermatology,
Universitat de Barcelona.

Antoni Surós i Batlló
Former Chief of the Digestive Department,
Hospital Universitari de Bellvitge,
l'Hospitalet de Llobregat, Barcelona.

Aureli Torné i Bladé
Specialist Consultor,Unitat de Ginecologia
Oncològica i Neonatologia (ICGON),
Hospital Clínic de Barcelona,
Barcelona.

Sandra Torra i Alsina
Specialist in Digestive System,
Secció de Digestología,
Hospital Parc Sanitari Sant Joan de Déu,
Universitat de Barcelona.

Anna Ureña i Lluveras
Specialist in Thoracic Surgery,
Hospital Universitari de Bellvitge,
l'Hospitalet de Llobregat, Barcelona.

Magí Valls i Porcel
Former Chief of the Gynecology
Department,
Hospital Universitari de Bellvitge,
l'Hospitalet de Llobregat, Barcelona.

Antonio Vidaller Palacín
Former Chief of the Internal Medicine
Department,
Hospital Universitari de Bellvitge,
l'Hospitalet de Llobregat, Barcelona.
Associate Professor in Medicine,
Universitat de Barcelona.

Núria Vilarrasa i García
Specialist in Endocrinology and Nutrition,
Hospital Universitari de Bellvitge,
l'Hospitalet de Llobregat, Barcelona.

Ignasi Viza i Puiggròs
Specialist in Otorhinolaryngology,
Servei d'Otorrinolaringologia,
Hospital Universitari Dexeus, Barcelona.

The life of each person is an adventure, a trip, a transit, in which occurs or might occur anything, good, bad, nice, not nice, success or failure, inspired situations or unexpected facts, coincidences, incidents, accidents. In any case, not everything what happens during life is pleasant and to add to that, bad things commonly appear by surprise, suddenly, in the worst moment and many times, in the worst conditions or circumstances. It is then when the overwhelmed person, without thinking about it, questions could come to head such as: what do I do now? How do I solve this problem? What decision should I take? When such situations occur is important to take the right decisions and know how to deal with this when being obliged to request the first aids.

First aid is defined as the treatment and care of an emergency that should be provided to a healthy person who has suffered an injury or accident, or a sick person who has had symptoms of certain serious disease. A first aid care or help must be an immediate and effective action as a previous step, or resistance situation, while it has been awaited to have specialized and specific medical attention.

First aids, as a result are a generic expression that refers to immediate, proper and provisional cares that are given to those injured or sick people before being properly treated by a competent health care professional. First aids are those measures or actions carried out that is done by the rescuer or helper in the same place and moment in which the incident has taken place with many time improvised means (materials, tools and remedies).

The first aids are therefore not medical treatments in the deepest sense of the word but some emergency actions which objective is to reduce or delay the effects of the injuries and stabilize the injured patient, so that these people might resist in the best conditions until the arrival of the medical assistance, without getting worse their situation and as far as possible, minimizing the suffering. This is what provides special importance to the first aids. It is important to highlight that the first actions which are taken, might be crucial for the evolution of the injured person, to the extent that a good decision of this first performance might depend many times the general state of the patient and over all, his or her future evolution, without excluding that well treated first aids may even save the life of the injured or sick patient.

When medical assistance has arrived, it will try to give solution to the problem by using all the means available that the medicine has, but in medical emergency situations, people who are near the injured are the ones who will have to act firstly and rapidly. That is why the first aids are very important.

In the light of the above, it should be added the social aspect, which is the greater importance in first aids: help any person, who has suddenly had a health problem, it is an obligation that nobody should forget.

As a main idea, when we talk about first aids, it is recommended to follow a logic strategy of actions which is well known as PAS, acronym that has the three initial letters of actions that should be followed in order to correctly attend the person who has suffered and important incident:

- Protect: before carrying out any action, it might be essential to assess the environment in order to find any risks that may affect the individual who needs help or other people who might have the same situation. The measures to be taken might depend on the accident place, although, in general protect with protective gloves, point the place of the accident and turn off the electrical and gas power in case of electrocution or intoxication.

- Warn. It is necessary to keep in touch as soon as possible with the nearest health assistance center by calling the medical emergency telephone number in order to have fast medical assistance, explain the case and receive instructions about the incident. That is why is absolutely useful to have a well visible, known and easy to reach place for everybody (at home could be behind the door, when travelling, next to the most important documents), a list with the most important emergency telephone numbers such as medical assistance, ambulances, firefighters, police, etc.

- Bring assistance. First of all, the helper should keep calm. Tell the injured person that the help is on the way to calm down. By the time the medical assistance arrives, it will be explained to the health assistants the lesions, all the circumstances and detected symptoms and everything that has been done to help the injured. The actions to follow, as a priority, will be decided and appropriate precaution will be taken in order not to make things worse the victim's situation and to speed up all that can help to solve the problem.

Whatever might be the circumstances which have caused the accident and the first aid that might be required to find the best solution, the main objectives that the first aids follow always must be clear:

- Keep the injured patient's life.

- Decrease the maximum possible risk of lesions or the effect after the accident.

- Avoid further physical or psychological complications.

- Help to the recovery.

- Make sure that the transfer of the injured patient to a health center might be in the best possible conditions, both the injured state as the rapidness, health attention and comfort of the transportation.

All the concepts that have been mentioned constitute the leitmotiv of this book.

As this could not be any other way, it is a book in which give importance to a series of certain characteristics: its practical aspect, an easy tool to use, with a rapid consultation, with concise and precise information. Depending on the end-use, the service that tries to provide the user and the circumstances in which the person might consult it, in any way it could be thought about a discursive book, with long text and endless expositions and lucubration, even if they could be very interesting. The words firs aids always suggest urgency, speed and immediacy. That is why the descriptions of the contents of this books are clear, concrete, expeditious and with an instant application.

Along these lines, the reader will see that is provided an important amount of tables, with almost telegraphic texts, multiple advices to fulfill with absolute promptness, actions to follow step by step, in order to the reader does not have to think about the what ant the how, but only be focused in the when, in other words, right now.

It is clear that the book could have been larger about the topics, moments and conditions which are subject to take into consideration about first aids, are countless. However, we are absolutely sure that the circumstances and type of accidents to which this book try to provide a response, are the most common, and as a result those situations that will guarantee a better use.

We hope, though, that this book might be one of the best recurrent when the necessity and urgency to a sudden problem might appear, and of course, that might be used when the nerves, despair, hurries, transfer and even some times a mixed up mind appear. Those are difficult and unpleasant moments in which a person, in addition of being altered, scared, despaired, and feels powerless and without knowing what to do. In case of somebody is in one of these situations, take this book, open it through the pages or pages which are appropriate to fulfill to the very detail, with the book in hand, we would say everything that is indicated about the case or circumstance in which the person is found. It is for sure, in addition of contributing to calm the patient, it will help the rescuer or helper to know what has to be done, without being scared to make mistakes in the attempt to make a successful respond to the particular situation.

I would like to finish this presentation with something that is obvious, although it might include a contradiction: despite of having tried to make every effort to put in the hands of the users a book that might be easy to consult, very useful and is characterized for being practical, our best desire is that never in life is going to be needed this book. In any case, although is difficult to have the luck of fulfilling our wish, just in case, we hope to provide with this book the best friend and best company that anyone might have when having an unexpected or difficult situation that may come as a surprise and we have never wished.

Jordi Vigué
Director of the Scientific Medical Team
Asklepios Medical Atlas

SUMMARY

FIRST AIDS

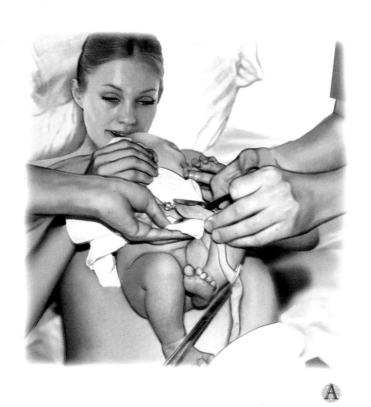

PREPARATION AND PREVENTION FOR AN EMERGENCY

First aid basic procedures

Cardiopulmonary resuscitation

- The cardiopulmonary resuscitation is an emergency procedure that is used as an effort for keeping manually the brain oxygenation until breathing and circulation can be restored when a cardio respiratory arrest occurs.
- The cardio respiratory arrest occurs when an individual's heart suddenly stops beating, for this reason the cardiopulmonary resuscitation is essential to maintaining oxygen flowing through the blood vessels and so that reach the tissues for keeping them working and avoiding after effects or even death.

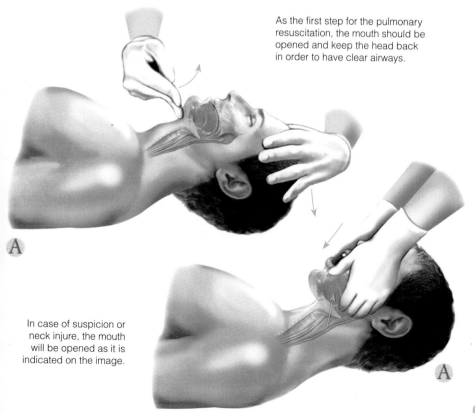

As the first step for the pulmonary resuscitation, the mouth should be opened and keep the head back in order to have clear airways.

In case of suspicion or neck injure, the mouth will be opened as it is indicated on the image.

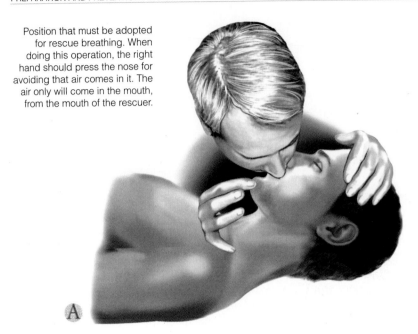

Position that must be adopted for rescue breathing. When doing this operation, the right hand should press the nose for avoiding that air comes in it. The air only will come in the mouth, from the mouth of the rescuer.

- The cardiopulmonary resuscitation is focused in the opening and keeping of the airway when tilting head back with the chin elevated and restore breathing through rescue breathing and circulation through chest compression.
- The cardiopulmonary resuscitation is indicated in three different situations:
  - When the victim is unconscious.
  - When the victim does not breath.
  - When the victim does not have pulse.
- When a person is unconscious, the priority is to ask for specialized medical aid and then, in order to assess and handle the situation, should be followed this sequence:
  - A. It indicates a reference to airway (A = airway). With the patient lying on the back on a firm surface, check with the fingers the presence of strange objects or loose teeth inside mouth, lean the head back and elevate the chin with the fingers of the other hand; look, feel and listen for breathing. In case of suspecting injury to the neck , open the airway by pulling the jaw towards you from both sides with each of your hands.
  - B. It refers to breathing (B = breathing). If the individual does not breathe but still has pulse, you have to close his nose by pressing it with the thumb and index fingers. While you have the airway open with a hand in the forehead of the patient, cover his mouth with yours after taking deep breaths. Provide two full breaths. Take deep air between each breath. Observe that after each breath should make the chest rise. In case of not being possible to provide air through the mouth because of a lesion, it should be given through the nose.
  - C. It refers to the circulation or compressions. If the breaths are not effective or from the beginning is not felt the pulse, chest compressions combined with breaths, should be restarted. Find the center of the patient's chest and begin 30 compressions, followed by 2 breaths. Continue repeating series of 30 compressions and two breaths until medical support arrives or until the patient moves or starts breathing.

HOW TO MAKE RESCUE BREATHING

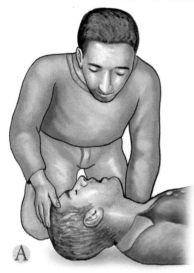

1 The affected person is softly placed face up and the head is leaned back. The jaw is opened.

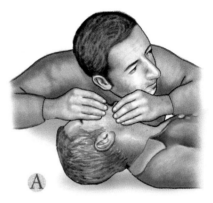

2 While you are blowing, check if the chest of the victim is inflated. Wait for five seconds, if the victim is an adult and three seconds if is a baby, and do this again.

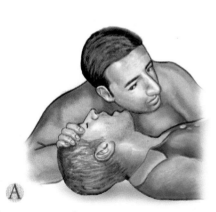

3 Verify if the victim is breathing and has pulse. If this is not the situation, rescue breathing has to be combined with the cardio respiratory resuscitation.

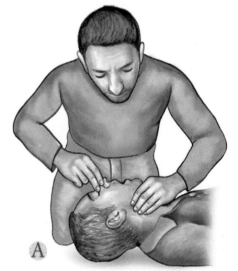

4 Cover the victim's nose with a hand and open the mouth. Cover the victim's mouth with the rescuer's mouth with and blow continuously.

RESCUE BREATHING		
ADULTS	CHILDREN	BABIES
• A breath every five seconds • 12 breathings per minute	• A breath every three seconds • 20 breathings per minute	• A breath every three seconds • 30-40 breathings per minute

POSITION ADOPTED FOR THE CHEST COMPRESSION

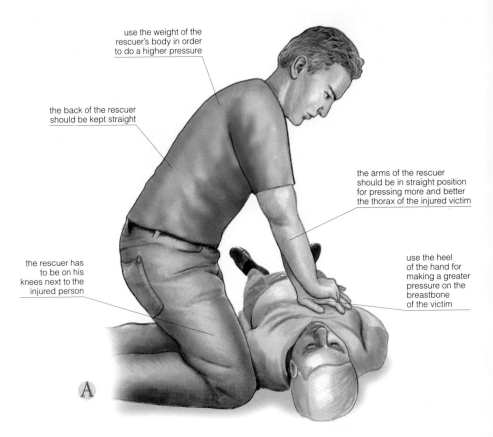

use the weight of the rescuer's body in order to do a higher pressure

the back of the rescuer should be kept straight

the arms of the rescuer should be in straight position for pressing more and better the thorax of the injured victim

the rescuer has to be on his knees next to the injured person

use the heel of the hand for making a greater pressure on the breastbone of the victim

A

THORAX COMPRESSION				
	ADULTS		CHILDREN	
A RESCUER	• 15 thorax compressions for every two breathings	• 80/100 compressions per minute	• 5 compressions for every breathing	• 80/100 compressions per minute
TWO RESCUERS	• 5 thorax compressions for every breathing and change of the rescuer's position.	• 80/100 compressions per minute	• It cannot be made	• It cannot be made

Taking the body temperature

- The temperature is measured with a thermometer. There are different types of thermometers for measuring the body temperature:
  - Mercury thermometer for the oral measure of the temperature.
  - Tympanic thermometer.
  - Rectal thermometer.

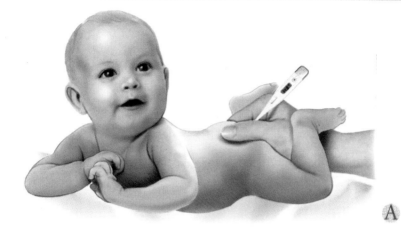

Taking of baby's temperature (anal), when is lying down.

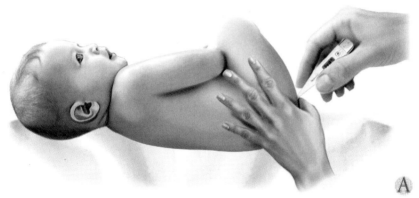

Taking of baby's temperature (anal), when is lying face up.

- The average body temperature in a healthy individual is about 37°C (98,6°F) +/- 1°C. The temperature registered with a rectal thermometer gives a higher reading in 1°C, in comparison with the temperature taken with an oral thermometer because of the airways and the mouth cooling for the inhaled air.

- In order to take the oral temperature, put the thermometer under the tongue for about 2 or 3 minutes if it is a glass (mercury) thermometer, or during 30 seconds (or until the sound indicates) in the case of a digital thermometer. Do not take the temperature ten minutes after having eaten any foods, after taking a shower or drinking liquids.'

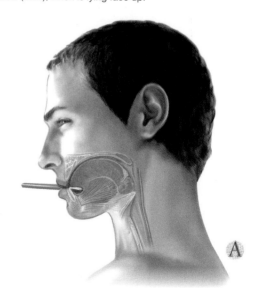

Oral taking of oral temperature. The thermometer should be placed under the tongue.

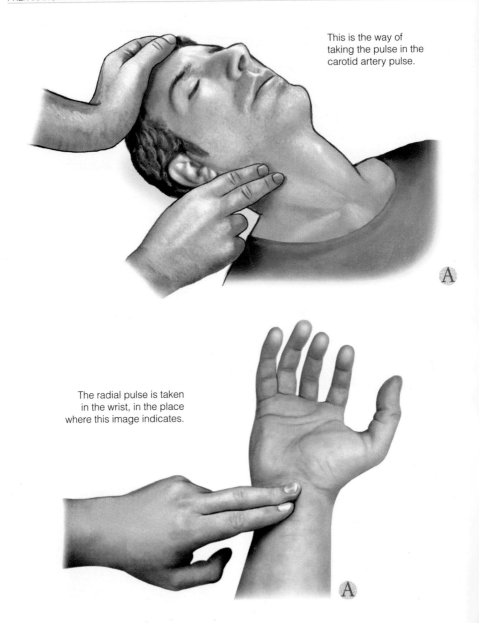

This is the way of taking the pulse in the carotid artery pulse.

The radial pulse is taken in the wrist, in the place where this image indicates.

- For the rectal temperature, place the small child face down on a stable surface, lubricates the thermometer with vaseline, spread the buttocks in order to see the rectum and introduce the thermometer approximately one centimeter. Once the thermometer has been placed, hold it and join the buttocks of the child during 2 or 3 minutes (for a mercury thermometer) or during 30 seconds (for a digital thermometer).

Identify the pulse

- The normal heart frequency (pulse) of an adult ranges from 60 and 100 beats per minute. The athletes or individuals who exercise regularly commonly have lower pulses of 60 beats per minute. For finding the pulse, use the three finger pads of one hand

ARTERIAL PULSES

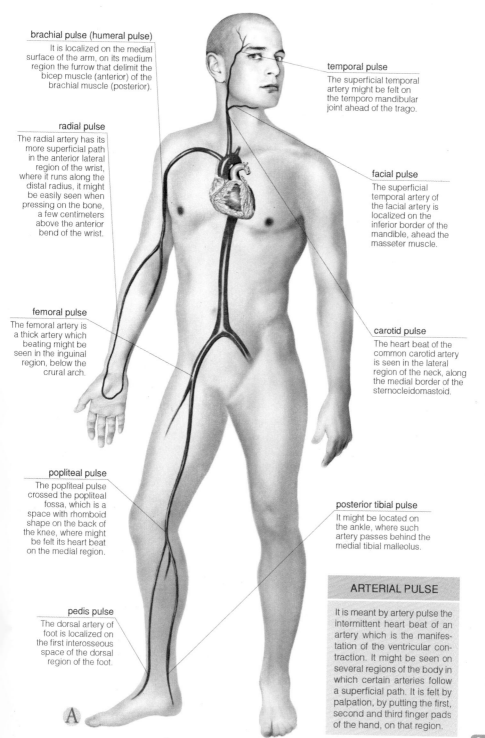

brachial pulse (humeral pulse)
It is localized on the medial surface of the arm, on its medium region the furrow that delimit the bicep muscle (anterior) of the brachial muscle (posterior).

radial pulse
The radial artery has its more superficial path in the anterior lateral region of the wrist, where it runs along the distal radius, it might be easily seen when pressing on the bone, a few centimeters above the anterior bend of the wrist.

femoral pulse
The femoral artery is a thick artery which beating might be seen in the inguinal region, below the crural arch.

popliteal pulse
The popliteal pulse crossed the popliteal fossa, which is a space with rhomboid shape on the back of the knee, where might be felt its heart beat on the medial region.

pedis pulse
The dorsal artery of foot is localized on the first interosseous space of the dorsal region of the foot.

temporal pulse
The superficial temporal artery might be felt on the temporo mandibular joint ahead of the trago.

facial pulse
The superficial temporal artery of the facial artery is localized on the inferior border of the mandible, ahead the masseter muscle.

carotid pulse
The heart beat of the common carotid artery is seen in the lateral region of the neck, along the medial border of the sternocleidomastoid.

posterior tibial pulse
It might be located on the ankle, where such artery passes behind the medial tibial malleolus.

ARTERIAL PULSE

It is meant by artery pulse the intermittent heart beat of an artery which is the manifestation of the ventricular contraction. It might be seen on several regions of the body in which certain arteries follow a superficial path. It is felt by palpation, by putting the first, second and third finger pads of the hand, on that region.

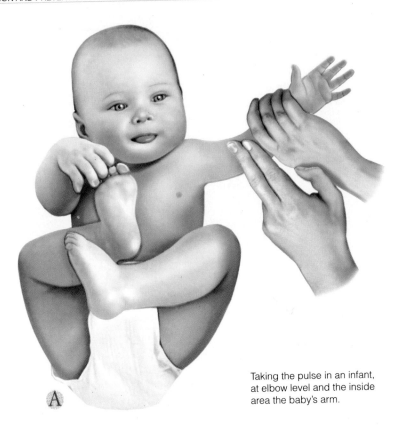

Taking the pulse in an infant, at elbow level and the inside area the baby's arm.

under the thumb in the in the palmar of the wrist. Once you feel pulses, count them during 60 seconds and this is the heart beating of the individual. The pulse measurement should be done when resting, with the patient seated, without having emotiona or physical incidents recently.

- In the children, the pulse is commonly faster. For taking the pulse, look for the beats under the left nipple or in the brachial artery, which is found between the elbow and shoulder, just in the middle of the arm. The pulse of an infant is frequently around 120 beats per minute, in a child from 1 to 5 years old is about 90 to 120 beats and the kids between 5 and 15 years old will be between 70 and 100 beats.

Identifying changes in the pupil reaction

- Pupils are the central and dark part of the eyes. An important difference in the size c the pupils (very big or very small) might be the clue of a medical problem.
- The identification of the pupils' size is essential for determining if their characteristic are appropriate or have any abnormality. What it should be specially taken into ac count is if both of the individual' pupils do not have the same size, because this coul suggest the presence of a serious trauma of the head, a cerebrovascular problem c a serious injury to an eye.
- The reaction of the pupils to the light is the ideal method for assessing the neurolog cal function related to the pupils. The normal and expected response is that pupi make smaller when exposing to the light, while when withdrawing light, the pup should recover their size.

CHANGES IN THE PATTERN OF THE PUPILS

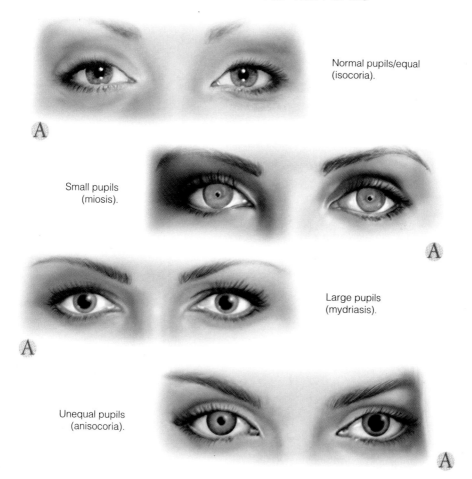

Normal pupils/equal (isocoria).

Small pupils (miosis).

Large pupils (mydriasis).

Unequal pupils (anisocoria).

First aid kit

• For an emergency medical care is useful to have to hand a first aid kit. The elements that an emergency kit should have are the next:
  - Sterile adhesive strips with different sizes.
  - Gauze rolls.
  - Sterile gauzes.
  - Micro porous adhesive tape.
  - Adhesive tape (plaster).
  - Scissors.
  - Toothless clamps.
  - Hydrogen peroxide.
  - Vaseline.
  - Thermometer.
  - Laminated cotton roll.

GENERAL RULES FOR PROVIDING FIRT AIDS

- Keep calm down.
- Identify yourself as a person trained in providing first aid, if this is your condition.
- Seek your own safety.
- Try to wear hygienic gloves.
- Do not moved the injured person if it is not necessary, or move the patient only what is needed for providing the first aids.
- Loosen clothing that makes pressure on the injured body, if it is necessary.
- Avoid giving drinks or food to the injured patient.
- Do not put alcohol on the injuries or on the injured person.
- Do not leave that the injured person might see the injuries or other people injuries.
- Remove curious people.
- Act if you are sure about what you are going to do. In case of doubt, restrain of acting.
- Act serenely, keeping quietness. From your attitude might depend the health or even the injured life. Avoid panic.
- Do not move next to the injured patient. In case of being alone, request for help.
- Give clear and precise orders.
- Do not leave the injured in less trained hands than yours.

- Cotton.
- Elastic bandages.
- Pain relievers or anti-inflammatories (acetaminophen, ibuprofen, naproxen).
- Hydrocortisone cream.
- Flash light.
- A jar of Saline solution.
- A jar of iodine.
- Sunscreen.
- Antihistamines (ceterizine, loratadine).

CUTTING TRAUMAS, BLEEDING AND AMPUTATIONS

Bleeding

- The blood in the human body flows through veins and arteries. The venous blood is commonly a little bit darker and has a slower flow that the arterial blood, which frequently has a bright red color and is expelled as a jet from the affected wounds. The arterial bleedings are more important because of the associated power and pressure, which implies loss blood at a higher speed and quantity. An arterial bleeding could be fatal.

External bleeding

- Doing tourniquets is an extreme measure that only could be used in situations that threaten the life of the affected individual or when the bleeding of a leg or arm is not

HOW TO CONTROL EXTERNAL BLEEDING

DIRECT PRESSURE

It is the elected method for the external bleeding control because of its high effectiveness. Sometimes it might cause pain development, however the continuous pressure is enough to control most of the external bleedings.

- Put a garment, towel, handkerchief or a pack on the wound and apply direct pressure through it.
- Keep a permanent pressure on the wound and raise the affected limb above the level of the victim's heart.
- Do not manipulate or alter the clots that are formed on the wound. If the blood is filtered through the garment with which pressure is applied, add another garment over the current garment and permanently keep the pressure.
- If bleeding stop or significantly decreases, make a pressure bandage on the wound. The bandage could be made with a tie or with a strip of clothing applied on the pack that was initially put to apply direct pressure of the wound. Do not remove the pack that was used to stop bleeding. The bandage should totally round the wound to be tied over the pack without making much pressure that might stop circulation, nevertheless it should be sufficiently firm in order to keep the pack on its position. Before finishing the tie, it should be made sure that circulation is maintained looking for a distal pulse (below) to the wound and bandage.
- Keep the limb of the wound elevated.

HOW TO STOP HEAVY BLEEDINGS IN A LEG

- Lay the victim face up.
- Press the heel of your hand over the central and front point of the union of the thigh with the groin and firmly press until bleeding is controlled. Do not exceed the pressure time because it could be harmful. If bleeding recurs when you take your hand away, renew the maneuver.

WHEN TO MAKE A TOURNIQUET

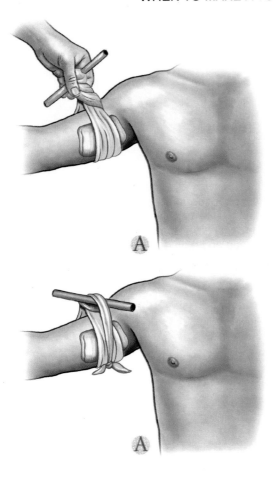

A tourniquet is a bandage that makes pressure on the arteries around the wound. Its function is to stop bleeding. It is a very dangerous technique that has to be carried out only in the next cases:

- When it has been tried to stop bleeding by using other techniques and it has not been possible. Before thinking about doing a tourniquet first has to be tried to stop the bleeding making strong pressure on the wound or on the points of blood pressure or by lifting the injured limb.

- If a limb has been amputated. Amputations commonly do not bleed immediately, but they could start at any moment, that is why a tourniquet has to be made for tightening at the moment of being necessary.

- If the bleeding is so severe that the life of the victim has been endangered.

- It should be reminded that a tourniquet would be considered as the last option for stopping a bleeding.

- Once is placed and tightened a tourniquet, never has to be removed by the rescuer because when releasing without medical precautions, the shock state gets worse and it even might cause the sudden death of the victim.

controlled with direct pressure or when applying direct pressure on the places previously mentioned because of the risk of losing a limb for the tourniquets in situations that are not indicated. In situations with a total or partial amputation, the risk of death is

THE TOURNIQUETS

- The tourniquet is an operation used to relieve a severe bleeding which cannot be stopped by the traditional system, through the compression of the whole blood vessels in a near circular area.
- The tourniquets only have to be used in the next cases:
  - When it is needed to attend more than one injured.
  - When a limb has been divided or crushed a limb.
- The tourniquets are placed above the elbow or above the knee, with a label in which is indicated the name and exact time of putting the tourniquet.
- Once the tourniquet has been placed, it should never be loosen.
- After doing the tourniquet, it should be seen with a label in which appears the name and exact time of putting it.
- It is important to remember that the tourniquets might imply risks: gangrene and death by auto intoxication.

PRESSURE POINTS IN ORDER TO BE TAKEN INTO ACCOUNT IN A TOURNIQUET

When an artery wound is placed in the neck or in the groin, the tourniquet is contraindicated, so that it will be necessary to make a manual compression until medical assistance arrives.

subclavian

The compression is made with the thumb in the subclavian and the rest of the hand in the back of the shoulder.

carotid

The compression is made with the thumb in the carotid and the rest of the hand in the back of the neck.

axillary

The compression is made with the thumb on the wound and the rest of the hand in the back of the armpit, without lifting the arm.

brachial

The compression is done with the thumb on the wound and the rest of the hand with a slight rise of the thumb.

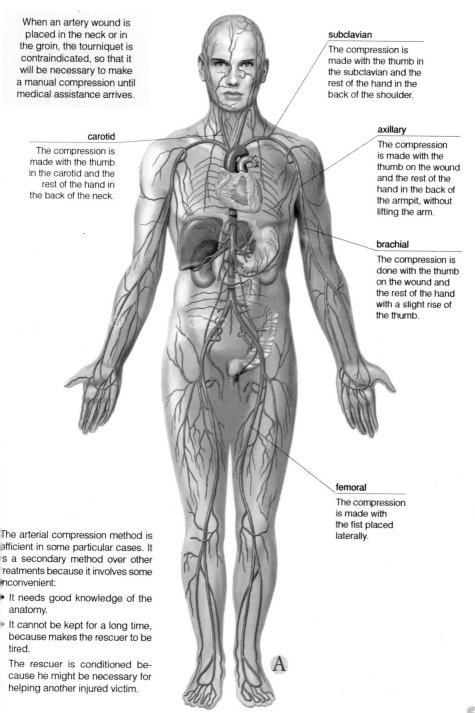

femoral

The compression is made with the fist placed laterally.

The arterial compression method is efficient in some particular cases. It is a secondary method over other treatments because it involves some inconvenient:

- It needs good knowledge of the anatomy.
- It cannot be kept for a long time, because makes the rescuer to be tired.

The rescuer is conditioned because he might be necessary for helping another injured victim.

HOW TO STOP HEAVY BLEEDING IN AN ARM

- Take the victim's arm feeling the bone in the middle of the armpit and the elbow with the thumb in the outside of the arm and the rest of the fingers inside with which could be felt the artery by pushingo.
- Close the hand trying to join the thumb with the rest of the fingers, making pressure on the bone until bleeding is stopped.

HOW TO DO A TOURNIQUET

- Get a strip of clothing, belt, tie, scarf or another material that is at least five centimeters wide and sufficiently long for completing two full turns to the wound and in order to tie it.
- Put the tourniquet over the wound, without touching it, complete two turns to the limb and tie it softly.
- Use a pen, pencil or another rigid or straight object in order to tie twice around it.
- Twist the pencil in order to tension the tourniquet until observing that bleeding stops.
- Write on a piece of paper the exact time in which was done the tourniquet.
- Stick the paper with the note to the patients, near to the tourniquet in order to be easily seen and identified by any person.

higher than the risk of definitely losing the limb, for this, is recommended to do a tourniquet. As it is possible, before doing a tourniquet, contact the emergency telephone number in order to get directions

Internal bleeding

- Though the internal bleeding might be a condition that seriously affects the health state of the individual, it not always an evident condition that might be easily identified. Internal bleeding could be suspected in individuals that have suffered an accident, categorical falls or traumas (knocks). Abdominal internal, chest and thigh bleedings are those that commonly get complicated.

SYMPTOMS OF INTERNAL BLEEDING

- Vomiting with the color of the coffee remains or completely red.
- Coughing up with bright fed and bubbly blood.
- Black of fresh stool.
- Pale appearance.
- Cold skin.
- Weak or rapid pulse.

- Distended abdomen.
- Fatigue, sleep.
- Thirst.
- Apprehension.
- Mental confusion.
- Disorientation.

HOW TO REACT IF INTERNAL BLEEDING IS SUSPECTED

- Contact the local emergency telephone number or as a priority, transfer the affected patient to the closest emergency services.
- If the individual does not breath, keep the airways open; restore breathing and circulation if necessary. *See the section about cardiopulmonary resuscitation*
- Do not give drinks of foods to the victim.
- Keep in contact and calm the victim.

ACTIONS FOR ENSURING LIFE OF THE INDIVIDUAL THAT SUFFERS AN AMPUTATION

- Call to the local telephone number for emergencies. Make sure that the injured patient breaths normally and be conscious. *See section for the management of the airways and circulation.*
- Treat and control bleeding.
- If vomiting has occurred in the victim, place the patient on his side on a solid surface or lightly turn his neck so that the chin is supported on the surface, you have to make sure that the individual does not have neck lesions (cervical). In case of any doubt, avoid moving neck and head.
- Once is assured the life of the individual, wash severely the affected limb with cold water (do not use soap or any other products).
- Put the amputated limb in a plastic bag with the care purposes that are described in the next figure.
- In the case that you carry the victim to the nearest emergency center, as soon as possible, call to the center about the accident and the presence of an injured victim with an amputation, in order to be prepared for this situation the emergency center.

ACTIONS TO PRESERVE AN AMPUTATED LIMB

- Rinse gently the amputated part with water or a saline solution (physiological saline solution), avoiding excessive rubbing. Do not apply soap or another substance, because it could seriously affect the integrity of tissues.
- Wrap the amputated part in gauzes or in a clean garment, previously soaked with water or a saline solution (physiological saline solution).
- Put the amputated part wrapped in gauzes or in a garment inside a plastic bag that as possible could be leak proof.
- Fully submerge the plastic bag in ice or in water with ice, preferably in a plastic container. It is important that ice is not directly in contact with the amputated part, because it could cause frostbites.
- Carry urgently the victim along with the amputated part to the nearest emergency center.

Amputations of parts of the body with small size

- The amputations of small parts of the body (fingers, ears, nose, penis) in general they present a better diagnosis than the amputations of bigger parts of the body such as complete limbs, in other words, they are easily saved and restored to the body. In order to keep safe and working an amputated part of the body, this should be kept in conditions where is guaranteed a temperature sufficiently cold for its preservation, ideally from 0° to 3° Celsius (38°F), in order to be restored to the body by the physician. If the part of the body is maintained to these temperatures, the muscle could be viable until 12 hours, while skin and bones might survive until 24 hours.
- In the cases of amputations, the first measure is to save the life of the victim and then restore the amputated part to the functionality. The individual who has suffered the amputation of a body part will have a massive bleeding and other conditions related to the trauma that should be assessed and managed. For this reason, it is essential to control the bleeding and then to be in charge as possible to preserve the amputated part.

BITES AND STINGS

Animal bites

- Animal bites may cause main infections, including rabies and tetanus, in addition may produce damage to the affected tissues for the bite. Dog bites represent the higher quantity of this type of accidents, while bats and small and medium size rodents are the main carriers and transmitters of rabies.

Human bites

- Human bites that alter the skin continuity, in other words, that might produce an open wound, require urgent medical attention. Human bites might produce important infections by bacteria or viruses that could cause contamination to the wound. Human bites in the hands might produce the loss of the fingers and hand function. Human

HOW TO AVOID ACCIDENTS CAUSED BY ANIMAL BITES

- Do not incite, provoke or suddenly stimulate an animal, especially when it is resting, sleeping or feeding.
- It is not recommended to have wild animals at home like if they were pets.
- Do not make sudden movements, neither sudden attitude with unknown animals.
- If an animal shows intention of attacking, keep calm and slowly move away from it.

WHAT TO DO FROM AN ANIMAL BITE

- Wash severe and immediately the wound with an iodine solution (1-5 %) or with soap and normal water for at least 5 minutes in order to reduce exposure and contamination for the microorganisms. Do not apply on the wound topical drugs, antiseptics or domestic medicines.
- Cover the wound with a gauze or sterile dressing. In case of not having any of them, cover with a clean cotton garment. When having active bleeding, apply continuous pressure during 5 minutes or until bleeding is stopped.
- Look urgently for medical attention, especially if the injury is on the face, neck or hands, because it will easily become complicated for infections that might even involve victim's life. In case of an amputation associated to the bite, bring the part of the body amputated to the emergency service according to the procedures that appear on the section of *Amputations* of this book.
- In the event of a suspicion that the animal associated to the accident might be the carrier of rabies, call to the police local service, emergency or animal care. It is important to capture and retain the animal that causes the accident in order to assess the presence of rabies that it may have; however do not try to capture the animal by yourself.

DOG BITES

- Most of the dog bites might be prevented, since they are caused because children bother dogs.
- Children that are near a dog, should always been watched.
- Avoid that the child approaches to unknown dogs.
- Adults should never leave a child alone with any dog.
- Never pet a dog without first letting it smell you.
- It is also important to teach the children that they do not have to get close to stray dogs or feed them.
- It is not recommended to approach to an animal that might have rabies or try to catch by your own.
- If you have a dog at home, it should be vaccinated periodically and request your friends that do the same.

WHAT TO DO IN CASE OF A DOG BITE

- Move away the animal with a stick or by agitating a big object and screaming the dog.
- Clean the superficial wounds with soap and water and apply an antiseptic.
- If you have latex gloves, it is better to wear them in order to protect from the exposure to the blood of another person.
- Cover the severe wounds and compress the bleeding with sterile gauze.
- Transfer the victim to a health care center in order to the physician decides if it is necessary any vaccine.
- When an individual is bitten by a dog, it is probable that the victim should take antibiotics, receive a reminder of the anti tetanus vaccine or rabies vaccination is needed.
- Bites and scratches in the hands or face of a child would likely become infected and it is necessary to be assessed by the physician.

bites are not considered the mode of transmission of the acquired immunodeficiency syndrome (HIV/AIDS).

Insect bites of sting

- Frequently the stings of the insects only cause local reactions, in other words, redness and swelling (edema) of the affected area. However, some times the stings might produce important allergic reactions, especially when the affected individual is allergic to the insect venom. The main insects which are related to the stings are the bees, paper wasps, hornets and fire ants.

WHAT TO DO FROM A HUMAN BITE

- Wash careful and immediately the wound with an iodine solution (1-5 %) or with soap and normal water for at least 5 minutes in order to reduce exposure and contamination for the microorganisms. Do not apply on the wound topical drugs, antiseptics or domestic medicines.
- Cover the injury with a gauze or sterile dressing. In case of not having any of them, cover with a clean cotton garment. In case of observing active bleeding, apply continuously pressure during 5 minutes or until bleeding is stopped.
- Look urgently for medical attention, especially if the injury is on the face, neck or hands, because it will easily become complicated for infections that might even involve victim's life. In case of an amputation associated to the bite, bring the part of the body amputated to the emergency service according to the procedures that appear on the section of *Amputations* of this book.

SYMPTOMS OF AN INSECT BITE OF STING

The insect stingers might generate some of the next symptoms. They generally appear in the bite zone as soon as it is presented or a few minutes later and they might last until 48-72 hours:

- Pain.
- Itching (pruritus).
- Burning discomfort.
- Sweling (edema).
- Redness.

WHAT TO DO FROM AN INSECT BITE OF STING

- In case that the insect has left the sting into the skin, try gently to remove it. It is recommended to use the edge of a paper, with a thin and blunt metal surface (knife, pocket knife, nail clippers, etc.) or with the nails. Avoid squeezing the skin and the sting because this will cause that venom from the sting insect might be released or might cause that such venom could be more rapidly absorbed.
- Wash carefully the affected area with soap and water. As a consequence of the insect bite sting do not break or explode the blisters because this could trigger a severe infection.
- Apply local cold through ice packs or ice which is wrapped in clothes in order to decrease absorption, spread, inflammation and pain of the venom.
- Give an oral antihistamine in order to reduce the symptoms (for example: loratadine, cetirizine).

- Although it is little frequent, sometimes a person might be affected by several bites with stingers. This situation does not necessarily affect the health's patient; however it requires urgent medical attention. The main observed symptoms related to this situation are the next:
  - Swelling of the affected area which appears immediately.
  - Headache.

SYMPTOMS OF AN ANAPHYLACTIC SHOCK

- Noticed swelling (edema) in areas of the body that are not affected by the insect bite such as eyes, lips, hands and tongue related to the swelling of the affected area.
- Coughing and wheezing.
- Generalized itching (pruritus).
- Difficulty breathing.
- Stomach cramps and abdominal cramps.
- Nausea and vomiting
- Anxiety
- Generalized weakness.
- Bluish discoloration of the skin.
- Collapse
- Loss of consciousness.

HOW TO REACT FROM AN ANAPHYLACTIC SHOCK RELATED TO A STING BITE

THERE IS NO EMERGENCY KIT	THERE IS EMERGENCY KIT
• Contact the local emergency number or urgently move the affected individual to the nearest emergency service. • If the individual does not breathe, follow the recommendations for keeping one of the airways and restore the circulation. (See the section about cardiopulmonary resuscitation).	• If the affected individual is not able to make a self-administration of the adrenaline injection, apply it by following the kit instructions. • Look for urgent medical assistance through the telephone of emergencies or carrying the victim to the closest emergency service.

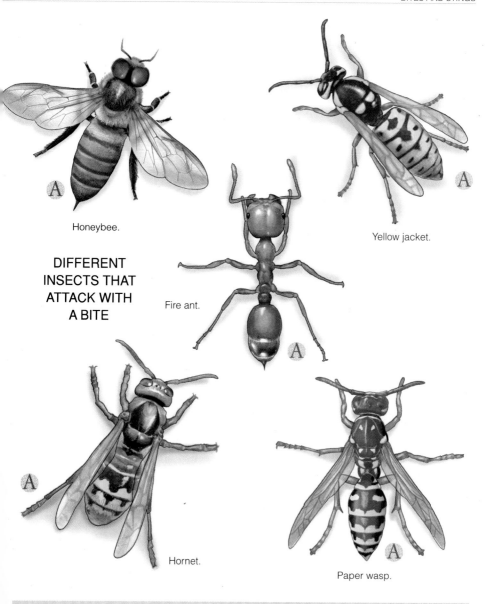

Honeybee.

**DIFFERENT
INSECTS THAT
ATTACK WITH
A BITE**

Fire ant.

Yellow jacket.

Hornet.

Paper wasp.

WHAT TO DO IN CASE OF A BITE

- Wash with water and soap the wound that has been caused by the insect.
- In case of bleeding, try to stop it by pressing the wound for a few minutes.
- Cover the wound with a sterile dressing.
- The severity of the bite depends on the next factors:
  - If the bite has been multiple, or if it has been on the face and/or neck, where the bite is more severe.
  - If the insect has bitten inside of the mouth might cause inflammation of the mucosa and difficulty breathing.
  - If the individual who has suffered a bite is allergic to insect bites, it could be cause an anaphylactic shock.
  - If the injured is a baby, a young child or an elderly person, the situation could be more difficult.

HOW TO AVOID BEE STINGING

- Avoid getting involved or handling honeycombs.
- Clean food remains, especially those which are outdoors and frequently remove trash from the house.
- Eliminate swarms by applying insecticide, particularly in the evenings, in the darkness, when the bees are inside and do not feel any activity.

HOW TO EXTRACT BEE'S STING

- Unlike ants and wasps that may use their sting, the bees, particularly the honey producing bees, embed their sting with toxic substances in the skin.
- The bee's sting contains inside a bag with toxic substances and germs, which are gently pumped by the skin after the bite.
- According to the popular belief, the stings of the bees should be removed from the skin by pitching the skin with the index and thumb fingers. However, this practice is not recommended at all because with this might be injected the rest of the liquid that is still in the sting.
- The right way to remove the sting is by scratching with an object that drags with a movement toward a side. The sting should be dragged carefully and in the same direction in which it penetrated the skin.
- When the sting has been removed, it might be applied a bag with ice on the sting area in order to relieve the inflammation and reduce the pain and the absorption of the venom.

- - Muscle cramps and muscle spasms.
- - Fever.
- - Dizziness, general weakness sensation.
- In view of this situation, follow the instructions for stings and call to the emergency service as soon as possible.
- Insect bite of sting might cause severe allergic reactions. They particularly appear in individuals that have been previously bitten and are sensitive to the current venom. The anaphylactic shock might be developed as a consequence of a bite and as a reaction from a sting and the related venom. The individuals that have developed a severe anaphylactic reaction prior to an insect bite of sting should be equipped with visible identification which classifies them as patients with that reaction and in addition with a kit for anaphylactic emergencies.

Spider bites

Black widow spider bite

- The black widow spider bite is particularly important in some groups of the population, especially in kids, elder people and chronically ill patients. This kind of spider appears in the hot or dry season, it might appear in the garbage, barns or places

HOW TO DEAL WITH A SPIDER BITE

- It should be applied a bag of ice on the zone of the bite in order to relieve the inflammation and reduce the pain and absorption of the venom.
- Apply a bag of ice and leave it for about ten minutes, remove the bag for ten minutes and do it again until the inflammation goes down.
- The injured patient must stay still.

SYMPTOMS RELATED TO THE BLACK WIDOW SPIDER BITE

- Swelling and redness located in the bite area.
- Acute and specific paina round the bite.
- Profuse sweating.
- Nausea and vomiting.
- Pain and abdominal cramps, rigid and tympanic abdomen within an hour of the bite.
- Muscle cramps and muscle contractures.
- Rigid thorax sensation (chest pressure) related to breathing and speaking difficulty.
- Generalized weakness.
- Facial swelling.

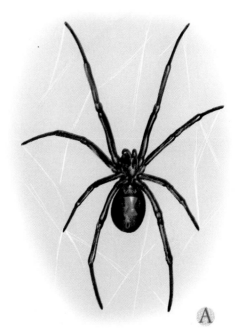

Black widow.

WHAT TO DO IN CASE OF A BLACK WIDOW BITE

- Go to the emergency room and inform about the bite.
- The specialist will prescribe medicines that will reduce the pain caused by the bite and muscle relaxants for the abdominal contractures.

with little light (garages, closets, etc.). Its net commonly has irregular form and it is particular and different to most of other kinds of spiders.

- The black widow might reach up to 2,5cm in length of its body and it is characterized by a reddish mark in the lower part of its body.

HOW TO REACT FROM A BLACK WIDOW SPIDER BITE

THE AFFECTED INDIVIDUAL DOES NOT PROPERLY BREATH	THE AFFECTED INDIVIDUAL PROPERLY BREATHS
• Contact urgently the local emergency telephone or transfer the affected person to the closest emergency service. • If necessary, keep the airway clear, restore breathing and circulation. *(See the section about cardiopulmonary resuscitation)*.	• Keep the bite area at a lower level of the heart of the affected patient. • Apply ice wrapped in a clean garment or cold compresses on the bite. • Keep the affected patient calm and silent. • Look for urgent medical attention transferring the affected individual to the closest emergency service. • If it is possible capture the spider in a safely way and take it with you, do it.

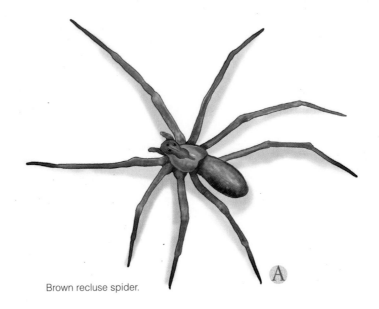

Brown recluse spider.

BROWN RECLUSE SPIDER BITE SYMPTOMS

- Feeling of stitch or bite at moment of the attack moment.
- Redness in the area of the bite, which progressively disappears observing the emergence of a blister.
- Intense pain which increases in severity in the period of 8 hours after the bite.
- Chills, fever, nausea, vomiting, shivers and widely erythema in the period of 48 hours after bite.
- Tissue destruction affected by the bite, characterized by the formation of an open ulcer which can persist during several months.
- Presence of blood in urine in the first day after the bite.

Brown recluse spider bite

- Brown recluse spiders are especially found in dark storerooms, frequently appearing in cupboards, attics, cabinets, piles of wood, under rocks or abandoned buildings. They are particularly active at night and it is very common that bites are shown while

HOW TO REACT ABOUT A BROWN RECLUSE SPIDER BITE

THE AFFECTED INDIVIDUAL DOES NOT BREATH ADEQUATELY	THE AFFECTED INDIVIDUAL IS BREATING ADEQUATELY
• Contact as a matter of priority emergency phones or transferring the affected individual to nearest urgency service. • Keep the air way open; restore breathing and circulation if necessary. *(See cardiopulmonary resuscitation section).*	• Keep bite area to a lower level of the heart of the affected individual. • Apply ice wrapped in clean clothing or cold compresses on the bite. • Keep the affected individual calm and quiet. • Look for medical assistance as a matter of priority transferring the affected individual to the nearest emergency department. If it is possible, capture the spider in a safe way and take it with you, do it.

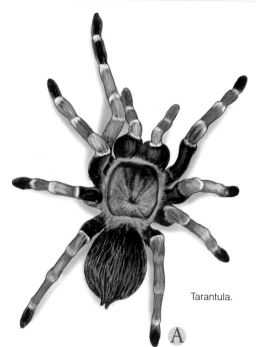

Tarantula.

individual sleeps when using sheets which have been stored during long time. This kind of spiders cause harmful effects especially in children and elder people, observing damage of main tissue around the bite therefore it is a priority to obtain medical assistance.

- Brown recluse spider is characterized by its brown color and the presence of a mark in violin front shape and upper part of its body.
- Presence of fever, blood in urine, widespread erythema or shivers implies a serious effect about associated health to bite, for this reason must be sought priority medical service in an emergency service.

Tarantula bites

- Tarantula bites do not use to have so serious effects on health as black widow spider or brown recluse spider; however, for its aspect more intimidating aspect the tarantula might generate more anxiety and fear. Tarantulas might reach lengths from 2,5 and 7,5cm and show a slower displacement and paused than the rest of spiders.

HOW TO REACT FROM TARANTULA BITE

- Remove the hairs of spider deposited in the bite area with adhesive tape or cellophane paper.
- Thoroughly wash the affected area with normal water and soap.
- Apply wrapped ice in clean clothing or cold compresses on the bite.
- Raise the affected area of the body for the bite above the heart level.
- In order to decrease the symptoms, give an antihistamine (loratadine, ceritizine), a pain reliever (acetaminophen) or anti-inflammatory (naproxen, ibuprofen, diclofenac), as long as the affected individual does not show adverse reactions to these medicines.
- If affected individual shows shortness of breath, general weakness, chest pain or loss of consciousness, contact your local number of emergencies or carry the person to the nearest emergency service.

HOW TO AVOID TICKS BITES

- At home, mow the lawn more frequently, remove grass clippings, pile wood in a dry and high place and remove frequently leaves and plant remains.
- When camping or hiking in wooded areas, wear shoes with socks, choose for long pants with wore socks on the bottom edge of the pants, and wear long sleeved shirts inside pants.
- Wear light-colored clothing with soft fabrics which adhere to the body, it will help to identify easily ticks and will avoid the contact of them with the skin.
- Review your body and clothing twice every day for discarding t ticks presence. Brush your body after hiking in wooded areas.
- Keep long hair in the back of the head; brush exhaustively the hair after hiking in a woodland area.
- Wash widely hair with shampoo after a hiking in a wooded area, wash promptly clothing after the same.
- Keep clothing and towels above the ground when camping or at the beach.
- Walk by paths very well bordered, mapped and clear.
- Consult to your veterinary with regard to products for prevention and treatment of ticks in pets.
- Use insect repelling to keep ticks away, especially the ones that contain N-dietil-metatolamida or permithrin.

- Tarantula is characterized by its large size (comparing to other spiders) and by its body covered with hair.

Ticks bites

- Ticks are arachnids which particularly grow up in woodland areas and are fed o animals as deers, rabbits and other rodents. Ticks have the potential to transmit to hu man beings organisms able to generate disease. Individuals who live near woodlands

HOW TO ACT FROM A TICK BITE

HOW TO REMOVE A TICK FROM SKIN	HOW TO REMOVE A TICK WHICH HAS BEEN INCORPORATED TO SKIN
• Do not touch the tick with your fingers; protect your hands with a pair of disposable gloves or with disposable tissue. Do not use a match or any other set fire element because it can cause that the tick introduces into the skin.	• Puncture delicately the external part of skin which contains the tick and carefully scrape it without cutting the tick with a blade of single edge previously sterile.
• In order to remove the tick, use tweezers, take and pull the head the nearest possible to skin. Avoid crushing or turning the tick body on the attempt. Push firmly and gently the tick in just only one piece, if tick loses head in the attempt to remove it, it could get in the skin.	• Clean the injury with antiseptic solution, ideally alcohol.
• If you are not sure or able to remove the tick consult with a doctor. If you remove it, you also have to consult with a doctor to confirm the tick has been completely removed.
• Kill the tick by putting and throwing it away into the toilet or applying it in a bottle with alcohol.	
• Wash your hands carefully with water and soap.	
• Clean the injury with antiseptic substance, ideally with alcohol.	
• Consult with a doctor to confirm that the treatment has been appropriate and to remove any part of the tick body that is still into the skin.	

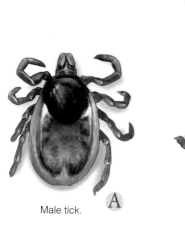

Male tick.

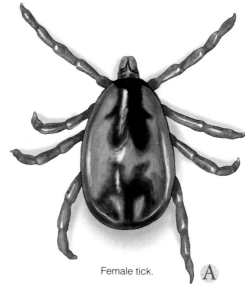

Female tick.

areas or camp or take walks in these areas are more likely to tick bites. Pets might bring ticks at home.

- Ticks are small, with medium-length of 3 mm. When biting a person or animal, the tick is adhered to skin, suck his blood and might extend their size from 5 to 7 times the original as product of sucked blood.

Bites at the sea

- Some marine life's bites are poisonous. The most common bites at the sea are the ones caused by aquamalas, jellyfish, scorpion fish and rays.

WHAT TO DO FROM AQUAMALA OR JELLYFISH BITE	
AQUAMALA BITE	AQUAMALA OR JELLYFISH BITE
• Remove urgently any tentacle which is adhered to skin through the use of gloves, wrap the hands in some clothing or using tweezers or pliers. Free tentacles (which are not adhered to aquamala) also can produce reactions/bites.	• Wash the affected area with sea water or vinegar (acetic acid) to deactivate poisonous cells. Do not use treated water or of the pipeline since this can activate cells and release the poison. • In order to remove the adhered cells to skin, apply shaving cream and shave the affected area carefully. You can also make a mix of sand or mud with sea water to rub the affected area. • In order to reduce the symptoms, apply hydrocortisone on the affected area or administer an antihistamine by oral way (loratadine, ceteicyne). • If affected individual shows difficulty for breathing, weakness or chest pain, contact the emergency local number or carry the victim to the nearest emergency service.

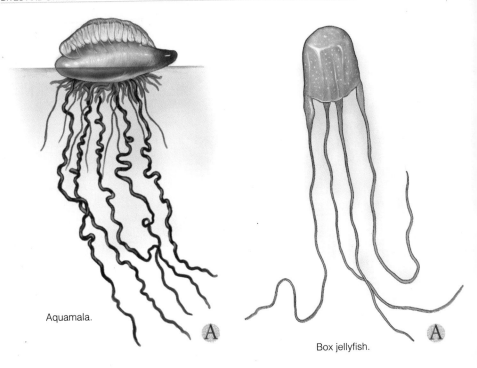

Aquamala.

Box jellyfish.

Bite by aquamala and jellyfish

- Jellyfish are poisonous even after dying. Aquamalas are commonly frequent in the American Atlantic Ocean, while jellyfish is frequent in the Pacific Ocean.

WHAT TO DO IN CASE OF JELLYFISH STING

- Do not clean the affected area with sweet water because it could cause a reactivation of the toxin. In order to wash the affected area, salty water, vinegar or water mixed with bicarbonate should be used.
- The affected area must not be rubbed with sand or with a towel.
- Apply cold to the affected area for about 15 minutes by using a plastic bag which contains ice. Direct ice should not be applied because being sweet water, it could be activated again the toxin.
- In order to relieve the pain, analgesics could be taken.
- If the injury state does not improve after ice has been applied several times or if the injured has fever, it is necessary to go to the nearest emergency centers.

ASSOCIATED SYMPTOMS TO AQUAMALAS AND JELLYFISH BITE

- Burn severe pain.
- Redness of the skin.
- Erithema and itchy of the skin.
- Cramps and muscle contractions.
- Nausea and vomiting.
- Difficulty breathing.

Important: If the bite affects more than half of the arm or the leg or if victim loses the awareness, contact as a matter of priority to the local emergency service or transfer as a matter of priority the victim to the nearest emergency service.

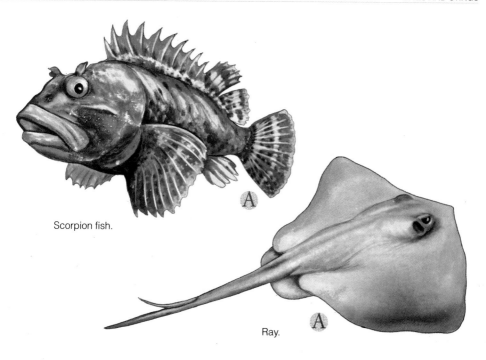

Scorpion fish.

Ray.

Scorpion fish bite (scorpionfish) and rays

- Stingray is a flat fish which is found in the bottom of tropical marine shallow water. Scorpion fish is a colored fish which is also found in tropical waters throughout the world. When are bothered, that is to say, when are stepping stingrays move swiftly their tails as defense mechanism, injecting poison present on it, usually in individual leg. Stingray tail and punzón are very powerful, being able to perforate plastic boots and diving cloths.

- Scorpion fish uses dorsum thorns as bite instruments, are able to simulate to be death when they really are not.

SYMPTOMS ASSOCIATED TO STINGRAY OR SCORPION FISH BITE

- Severe pain in the affected area.
- Nausea, vomiting and abdominal cramps.
- Tachycardia, rapid pulse, palpitations.
- Dizziness.
- Contractures and muscle cramps.

HOW TO ACT TO STINGRAY OR SCORPION FISH BITE

- Put the affected area of bite in hot water (45°C, 113°F) but not too hot that might cause a burn. Take the victim to the nearest emergency center with the part of the affected body immersed in the water; the required time is from 30 to 90 minutes to deactivate poison through this method.

- As far as possible, keep immobile the affected area.

- If it is not possible to take the victim to the emergency service, keep the affected area in hot water at least during 90 minutes and look for medical help as soon as possible.

29

SCORPION BITES

- Most of these injuries are accidentally produced, when stepping or having contact with the scorpion.
- After a scorpion bite commonly might appear:
  - Severe pain in the area.
  - Burning sensation that may disappear 48 hours later of having the bite.
  - Local inflammation.
  - The skin changes the color on the bite area, which normally gets a lighter color.
  - Restlessness and irritation.
  - General discomfort.
  - Fever
  - In the most severe cases: chills, shaking and rarely, shock.
- The severity of the bite depends on the age, height and weight of the affected victim and also if has received one or more bites.
- The venom of the scorpions is similar to the one of the bees and wasps.
- The scorpion bite may be particularly more severe for children because the venom of the scorpion contains neurotoxins and the nervous system is not completely mature, and as a result, is more sensitive to the action of the neurotoxins.
- In case of having a scorpion bite:
  - Clean and disinfect the bite.
  - Apply local cold and keep the limb high, if it is possible.
  - It has to be applied a bag with ice on the area of the bite in order to relieve the inflammation and reduce the pain and venom absorption.
  - Leave the applied bag for about ten minutes and remove it for ten minutes. Repeat the same operation until reducing the inflammation.
  - The injured should stay still.
  - It will be administered an analgesic/anti-inflammatory.
  - Anti tetanus prophylaxis.
  - Control the vital signs of the patient until having medical support.
  - At the hospitals there is anti venom for these cases.

Scorpion bites

- Some species of scorpions are more poisonous than others. The scorpion bites should be treated and assessed, especially in kids because the high potential of complications that might cause. The scorpions commonly hide under wooden branches and

SYMPTOMS RELATED TO THE SCORPION BITE

- Severe and burning pain in the affected area.
- Nausea and vomiting.
- Abdominal pain.
- Tingling and numbness in the affected area.
- Spasms of the jaw muscles, making difficult the oral opening.
- Tachycarcia, heart palpitations.Taquicardia, palpitaciones.
- Blurred vision
- Spasms and twitching of the affected muscles.
- Seizures.
- Coma.

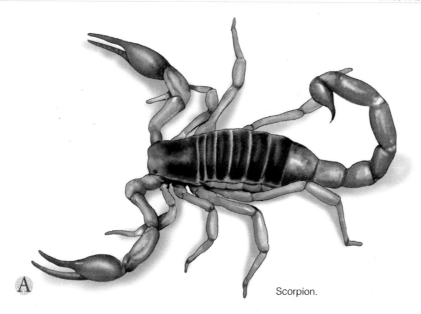

Scorpion.

HOW TO REACT FROM A SCORPION BITE

IF THE VICTIM DOES NOT BREATH	IF THE VICTIM BREATHES
• Contact urgently the emergency telephone. • Keep the airway opened; restore breathing and circulation if necessary.	• Keep the affected area by the scorpion bite at a lower level of the heart. • Apply wrapped ice in any garment or apply cold compresses on the affected area. • Keep the victim relax and quiet. • Look for medical attention as a priority and transfer the victim to the closest emergency service.

cracks on the ground, and they are usually found in desert areas of North, Central and South America. The scorpions are more active and their bites take place particularly in hot nights.

Snake bite

• The most important aspect to determine after a bite is if the snake is poisonous or not. The main poisonous snakes are the rattlesnake, water moccasin, copperhead and coral.

• The snake bites commonly take place in hot day, affecting legs and then arms.

MEASURES FOR AVOIDING SCORPION BITES

• Remove all the remains of wood, dead wood and pyre burning remains that are near your house.
• Install your camp far away from the Wood remains.
• Make sure of wearing shoes at every moment in areas of possible habitat of the scorpions.
• When camping, vigorously shake clothes and sheets before using them.

SNAKE BITES

- Snake bites are one of the most frequent and dangerous accidents that might be produced in the rural area.
- The snake is generally a quiet animal and is little aggressive, and, when it hears a noise, runs away. The snake only attacks if has been threatened or somebody is on its way.
- The snake bites commonly cause wounds, and as a result, they should be treated as such.
- Most of the snakes bite in the limbs.
- It is generally very difficult to know what kind of snake has attacked the victim since they fled from the place where the bite has taken place.

WHAT TO DO IN CASE OF A SNAKE BITE

- It is necessary to step back as soon as possible from the snake that has caused the bite. They commonly disappear rapidly; somehow it should not be forgotten prevention because other bites generally have more venom than the first one.
- Try to calm down the individual who has suffered a snake bite.
- Lay down the victim on the floor and try that does not move to avoid that blood circulation increased the poison absorption.
- Wash the wound with soap and water.
- Apply ice on the wound.
- If the bite has been caused on a limb, try to immobilize it.
- Remove rings or any other bead or object that compress because the affected area might become swollen.
- Take the victim to the emergency room.

- Poisonous snakes are mainly characterized for having a triangular head and also deep nostrils (venom sacks). The eyes are commonly enlarged instead of being rounded. The coral snake is the exception to this rule, because is poisonous and does not have a triangular head and also rounded eyes. The poisonous snakes are also characterized by the presence of fangs. The coral snake belongs to the family o cobras, it has red, yellow and black ring, it is a characteristic the presence of a yel

SYMPTOMS OF A NON-POISONOUS SNAKE BITE

- Moderate pain.
- Swelling of the affected area.
- Moderate bleeding.

HOW TO PROCEED FROM A NON-POISONOUS SNAKE BITE

- Keep the affected area below heart level.
- Remove from the patient, rings, watch or other jewelry.
- Wash carefully the wound with soap and water. Do not apply ice on the wound.
- Cover the wound with a bandage or a clean sterile dressing.
- Look for medical attention; it is possible that the patient requires a vaccination against tetanus and the use of antibiotics.

CHARACTERISTICS OF THE SNAKES

POISONOUS

NON POISONOUS

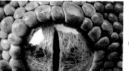

enlarged pupil (except the coral snake)

round pupil (except the coral snake)

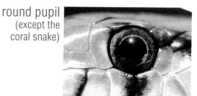

eyes

many figures with rhombuses, triangles

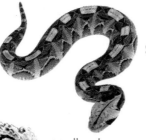

skin

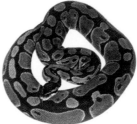

colors without geometrical figures

small and rough scales on the head (except the coral snake)

smooth plaques on the head (except the coral snake)

texture

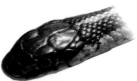

triangular head (except the coral snake)

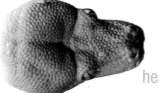

elongated head (except the coral snake)

head

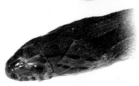

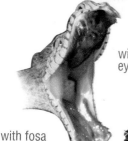

with front eyeteeth

eyeteeth

without front eyeteeth

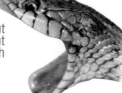

with fosa loreal

 short

tail

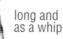 long and as a whip

without fosa loreal

nocturnal, twilight coral

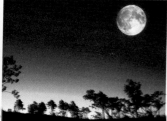

activity

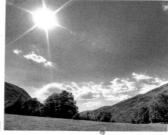

 diurnal

SYPMTOMS ASSOCIATED WITH THE BITE OF THE RATTLESNAKE, COTTONMOUTH AND COPPERHEAD SNAKE

- Severe pain.
- Swelling that rapidly dissapears.
- Loss of the normal skin color around the bite area.
- General weakness.
- Nausea and vomiting.
- Difficult breathing, lack of air sensation and chest pressure.
- Blurred vision.
- Convulsions
- Numbness of arms and legs.
- Redness of the affected area caused by the bite.

low ring (thinner than the other ones), separating the red rings from the black ones. It is also a characteristic of the coral its black nose and smaller size in comparison to the other poisonous snakes. Its venom is highly toxic and, unlike the other poisonous snakes, the coral commonly bites several times and chew the victim's tissues, the rest of the snakes tend to bite and then release immediately the victim.

- As it is possible, catch and kill the responsible snake of the bity without altering its head and take it to the medical emergency service. Handle with care the snake because the venom that is still present on its head might be active and harmful until

HOW TO ACT FROM THE BITE OF THE RATTLESNAKE, COTTONMOUTH AND COPPERHEAD SNAKE

IF THE INDIVIDUAL DOES NOT BREATH PROPERLY

- Contac the emergency telephone number or as a priority, take the patient to the closest emergency medical center.
- Keep open the airways; restore the airway and circulation in the case of being necessary. *(See the section about cardiopulmonary resuscitation).*

IF THE INDIVIDUAL IS BREATHING AND THERE IS A KIT FOR THE MANAGEMENT OF A POISONOUS SNAKE BITE

- Use the suction devices of the kit in order to remove the venom and body fluids associated to the bite place, preferably a few minutes after the bite.
- Keep the victim calm and quiet in order to reduce blood flow which decreases the spreading poison.
- Remove from the patient rings, watch or any other jewelry.
- Wash carefully the affected area with water and soap. Do not apply ice because it might damage the affected tissues.
- Cover the wound with a bandage or clean sterile dressing.
- Immobilize the affected limb and keep it lower than the heart. Do not allow that the victim walks at least it would be absolutely necessary.
- Give the patient small sips of water if there is no difficulty for swallowing. Do not give any liquid or food if the victim is having nausea, vomiting, convulsions or with impairment of consciousness.
- Look for urgent medical attention by taking the victim to the closest emergency medical service. As possible, previously report to the emergency center about the type of bite and the snake characteristics so that they may be ready with the serum in order to counteract the venom effects.

SEVERAL SNAKES THAT ATTACK WITH BITE

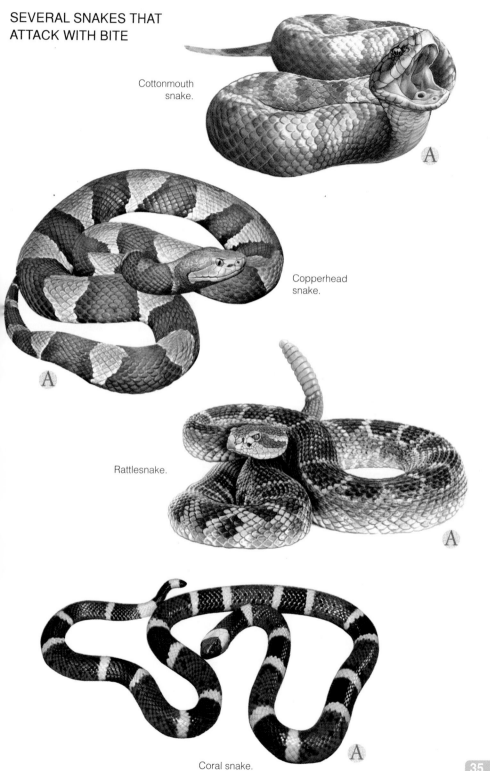

Cottonmouth snake.

A

Copperhead snake.

A

Rattlesnake.

A

Coral snake.

A

SYPTOMS ASSOCIATED TO A CORAL SNAKE BITE

- Moderate pain and swelling around the bite place.
- Blurred vision.
- Droopy eyelids.
- Have difficulty for speaking or swallowing.
- Dizziness.
- Profuse sweating.

- Nausea and vomiting.
- Have difficulty breathing.
- Paralysis.
- Joing pain.
- Confusion.
- Increased salivation.

HOW TO ACT FROM A CORAL SNAKE BITE

IF THE INDIVIDUAL DOES NOT BREATH PROPERLY

- Contac the emergency telephone number or as a priority, take the patient to the closest emergency medical center.
- Keep open the airways; restore the airway and circulation in the case of being necessary. *(See the section about cardiopulmonary resuscitation).*

IF THE INDIVIDUAL IS BREATHING AND THERE IS A KIT FOR THE MANAGEMENT OF A POISONOUS SNAKE BITE

- Use the suction devices of the kit in order to remove the venom and body fluids associated to the bite place, preferably a few minutes after the bite.
- Keep the victim calm and quiet in order to reduce blood flow which decreases the spreading poison.
- Remove from the patient rings, watch or any other jewelry.
- Wash carefully the affected area with water and soap. Do not apply ice because it might damage the affected tissues.
- Cover the wound with a bandage or clean sterile dressing.
- Immobilize the affected limb and keep it lower than the heart. Do not allow that the victim walks at least it would be absolutely necessary.
- Give the patient small sips of water if there is no difficulty for swallowing. Do not give any liquid or food if the victim is having nausea, vomiting, convulsions or with impairment of consciousness.
- Look for urgent medical attention by taking the victim to the closest emergency medical service. As possible, previously report to the emergency center about the type of bite and the snake characteristics so that they may be ready with the serum in order to counteract the venom effects.

one hour after being dead. If it is not possible to catch the snake, remember and write down its characteristics in order to mention at the moment of visiting the medical office.

BONE, JOINT AND MUSCLE INJURIES

Fractures

- The break or loss of the normal bone continuity is called fracture. The fractures might be open or closed fractures. In the closed fractures, there is no exposure of the bone through the skin, in other words, the skin maintains its normal integrity.

- In an open fracture, it is seen an open injury that is directly extended to the fractured bone. The open fractures are considered with a higher medical importance, because are associated to an increased bleeding and a higher probability of associated infections.

- Neck fractures or the spinal cord have to be carefully observed if the victim has lost consciousness, if has suffered a trauma to the head, in case of having a severe neck pain or if has a tingling sensation, paralysis or limitation for moving arms and legs. In case of any fracture, especially neck fractures, initially do not move the victim, with the

SYMPTOMS THAT MAKE YOU SUSPECT A FRACTURE

- The victim has suffered a fall or listened to a cracking sound in a bone.
- The area of the injury has an increase of the tenderness and severe pain, particularly when moving or touching it.
- The victim has difficulty for moving the affected zone.
- The affected area by the hit, presents unusual or little natural movements.
- The victim has a rubbing or friction sensation of the bone in the affected area.
- The affected zone by the trauma shows a significant inflammation (swelling).
- It is observe deformity in the affected zone.
- The area affected by the hit, shows discoloration or a bluish tone.
- The shape or length of the affected bone is observed different to the same bone of the other side of the body.

SYMPTOMS OF THE FRACTURES

- Severe pain. The pain is commonly placed in the place of the fracture and increases when it is tried to move the affected limb or when making pressure, however light.
- The affected limb must not be moved due to the own fracture and the pain that it might cause.
- Roughness sensation, caused by the rub of the fractured bones.
- Deformation and swelling of the affected limb.
- Hematoma. It is produced by the broken vessels broken around the fractured bone.
- Fever. It might appear in young people and in case of main fractures, without infection. It also may reappear during the reabsorbing process of the hematoma.

TYPES OF BONE FRACTURES (I)

BONE FRACTURE

A fracture is a broken bone, and is generally caused by trauma or, sometimes, a violent contraction of the muscles that are inserted into the fractured bone, and its also considered a bone disease. Bone fracture is accompanied by more or less severe injuries to adjacent soft tissues. The fractures are classified and named according to their severity, the shape and position of the fracture line or the name of who discovered it first. The fractures shown below are the most frequent.

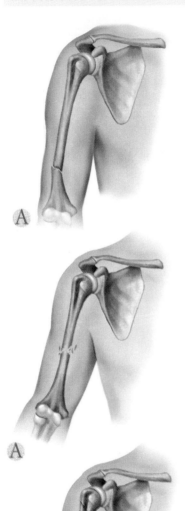

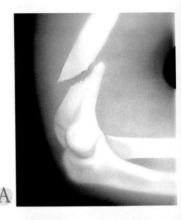

exposed fracture (or open fracture)

The broken ends of bone makes protrusion, through it, while in a simple fracture there are no protrusion.

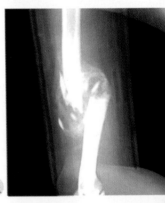

comminuted fracture (or broken into pieces)

Complete fracture in which bone splinter in the impact place and between the two main bone fragments resulting from the break, there are other smaller pieces. It usually occurs as a result of forced dorsal flexion of the hand, usually trying softening a fall and extending the upper extremity.

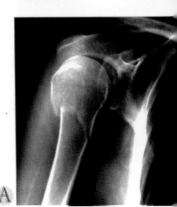

impacted fracture (or fracture by impact)

Is a fracture in which one of the fragments is introduced into the spongy bone of the other, as embedded in it, usually caused by a fall less important on the hand, where the force is transmitted through the upper arm.

TYPES OF BONE FRACTURES (II)

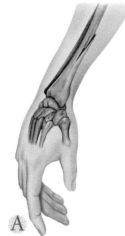

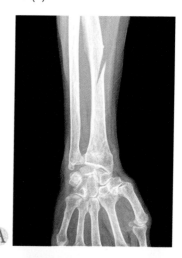

greenstick fracture

Incomplete fracture in which one side of the bone is fractured while the other is curved. It happens only in children, because their bones are not yet fully ossified and contain more organic material than inorganic. This fracture is produced by bending and characterized by permanent bending of the bone, which can be angled, and by the existence in his convexity of an incomplete fracture that effect the cortex. On the concave side remains flexed but not broken.

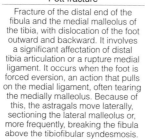

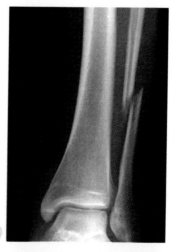

Pott fracture

Fracture of the distal end of the fibula and the medial malleolus of the tibia, with dislocation of the foot outward and backward. It involves a significant affectation of distal tibia articulation or a rupture medial ligament. It occurs when the foot is forced eversion, an action that pulls on the medial ligament, often tearing the medially malleolus. Because of this, the astragals move laterally, sectioning the lateral malleolus or, more frequently, breaking the fibula above the tibiofibular syndesmosis.

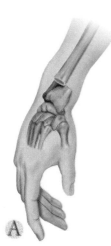

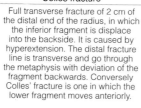

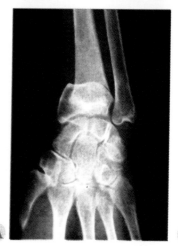

Colles fracture

Full transverse fracture of 2 cm of the distal end of the radius, in which the inferior fragment is displace into the backside. It is caused by hyperextension. The distal fracture line is transverse and go through the metaphysis with deviation of the fragment backwards. Conversely Colles' fracture is one in which the lower fragment moves anteriorly.

HOW TO DEAL WITH A SUSPICION OF FRACTURE

A CLOSED FRACTURE IS SUSPECTED	AN OPEN FRACTURE IS SUSPECTED
• Follow the immobilization specific steps for the affected zone of the trauma.	• As a first step, contact the nearest emergency local number. • Cut away any clothing that is close to the wound, leaving a space without clothing around the wound. • Without any reason try to insert the bone or exposed tissues to the wound. • Do not wash the wound; neither insert any device or gIve medicines. • Apply direct pressure on the wound with a clean garment or with a sterile dressing in order to reduce or stop bleeding. • Cover the whole wound, including the exposed bone, with a bandage or clean garment.
• If the fracture causes severe symptoms, contact your closest emergency number or take the victim to the nearest emergency service.	• Immobilize the joint or affected zone in case of not having medical or paramedic help. Always immobilize the joint over and below the affected area. • Handle or softly take the victim in order to avoid displacements or complications of the fracture. • Do not give the victim any foods or drinks.

exception when there is a situation of life threatening (fires, risk of explosion, presence in a zone of high vehicle traffic, etc.).

• In case of being indispensable to move the victim, as a priority, immobilize the affected area.

• In case of traumas into the water, and it is suspected a neck fracture, do not move the victim until immobilizing the whole spinal column with the help of a plank of wood or another rigid structure. In case of being necessary to move the victim, take the patient from the armpits or legs, always keeping the alignment between the neck and the rest of the body.

WHAT TO DO IN CASE OF A FRACTURE

Generally fractures have a fast and easy recovery. If there is a fracture, it is very important to immobilize the affected area and follow a series of advices for the right recovery:

• Relieve the pain by applying ice packs or towels.

• Keep the injured person in the most comfortable position but avoid the slightest movement.

• Do not try to replant the broken bone.

• Loosen clothing although should not be tried to take clothing off. This should be done by specialized personnel.

• Take the injured person to the nearest emergency center. If appropriate, an ambulance should be called or transfer the injured supporting the wounded limb on a splint.

• If the wound is open, it should be washed with running water and if possible, cover it with sterile gauze.

• Do not probe the wound.

• The injured should be asked if is vaccinated against tetanus in order to be able to prevent an infection.

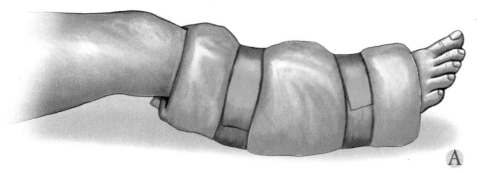

Immobilization of the ankle with a pillow.

Immobilizations

- The main objective of doing an immobilization is to avoid that the affected joint or bone might freely move. When immobilizing a fracture is possible to reduce the pain and there is a possibility that the fracture worsens or displaces. Life vests might be used to apply around the knees or ankles when these are the joints affected by a fracture. As possible, immobilization should be extended from the joint above and until the joint below the fracture.

- Immobilizations should be fixed in order to be stable; they could do it by using ties, strips of cloth, handkerchiefs, ropes or any other similar material. The fixation of the immobilization with these elements has to be very firm to be maintained in its position, because might alter or decrease the circulation until the affected zone and structures and distal tissues to the affected zone.

- When after the immobilization of the affected zone, it is observed a change in the skin coloration, numbness sensation or difficulty for moving the limb, the pressure or the strength of the immobilization should be reduced.

- It must always be looked for a distal pulse to the place of the immobilization. in order to make sure that circulation is appropriate. In case of not feeling or palpating the pulse, be sure of decreasing the tension of the fixation.

- If any fracture is suspected, it should be assessed urgently by the physician. After immobilizing the fracture, take urgently the victim to the nearest emergency room service.

Ankle fractures

- The limitation for walking, supporting or moving the ankle suggests a fracture of this joint. In case of the presence of bluish coloration, numbness sensation, limitation or difficulty for moving the fingers, take urgently the victim to the nearest emergency

THINGS THAT COULD BE USED FOR MAKING LIMB IMMOBILIZATIONS	
• Wooden boards.	• Pillows.
• Straight wooden sticks.	• Rolled sheet sets.
• Brooms.	• Skis.
• Cardboard.	• Paddles.
• Rolled newspapers or magazines.	• Umbrellas.

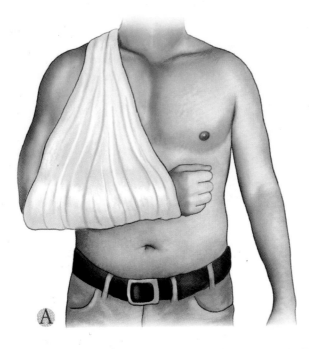

Immobilization when an arm fracture is suspected.

HOW TO DEAL WHEN AN ANKLE FRACTURE IS SUSPECTED

- Keep the victim lying down.
- Remove the victim's shoes.
- Put strips of cloth under the victim's leg. Put a pillow on the strips of cloth and under the ankle and covering the whole calf and be sure that has the appropriate length in order to wrap the whole leg and its edges in the front of the leg.
- Wrap the leg with the pillow fixing it in the front.

room service. If the individual is stable and do not have the above symptoms, proceed to the immobilization of the ankle.

Arm fractures

- If the pulse cannot be detected in the wrist, if it is observed movements limitation of the wrist, fingers or forearm, if the victim has numbness sensation in the fingers of the hand of the affected arm, the priority should be to carry the victim to the closest

HOW TO DEAL WITH AN ARM FRACTURE

- Put an element on the affected underarm which provides a mattress like effect, it might be used a foam or another soft material that cushions the joint. Place the affected arm in the side of the victim, with the lower arm at a right angle on the chest.
- Carry out an immobilization with a cushioned soft material on the lateral part of the arm. You might use a newspaper or rolled magazines. Place the newspaper in the upper and lower part of the fracture. Provide support to the arm with a sling that will be fixed to the neck.
- Keep the immobilization in the right position, by fixing it with a sheet that will be tied to the opposite side of the victim's chest, under the armpit.
- Keep the victim seated while is carried to the closest emergency room service.

HOW TO WRAP AN ANKLE

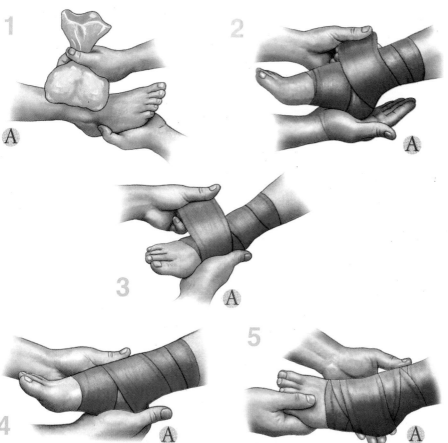

- It should be started by putting two sticking plasters on the leg, below the twins, and close them at the front of the leg. It always has to be taken into account that the leg does not have to be pressed excessively in order not to hamper the leg circulation.

A third bandage of plaster is put, this time below the first and toe.

It has to be placed a third sticking plaster in a U shape, which will have to be fixed to the first one, passing below the heels.

This U shape plaster has to be fixed to the ankles. It has to be adhered conveniently, making a little pressure with the fingers, trying not to hurt the ankle.

A bandage in a C shape is put, which surrounds the calcaneous tendon and goes to the bandage that surrounds the first and last toe. After that is adhered to this zone.

It is repeated once again the bandage of figure 3, but this time moving the position of the sticking plaster a little bit forward.

It is repeated the bandage of the figure 5. It is repeated the action of the last two figures until

three U shape bandages and three C shape bandages are gotten.

- It is placed another tape strip that will go from the external ankle to the internal heel. The part of the bandage that passes through the external ankle will cover the one that comes from the internal heel. This sticking plaster will be fixed to the first piece of plaster that is shown in the figure 1. It is repeated this action the other way around, putting a sticking plaster that will go from the internal to the external ankle.

- Bandages are placed as it is shown in the figure 1, but slightly moved down, in order to stabilize those bandages that have already been fixed.

- This operation is repeated, moving each piece of plaster a little bit down until is reached the instep of the foot.

- It is put another bandage as it is shown in the figure 2 in order to ensure those that have just been fixed.

- All of the sticking plasters are pressed in order to make sure they are well fixed.

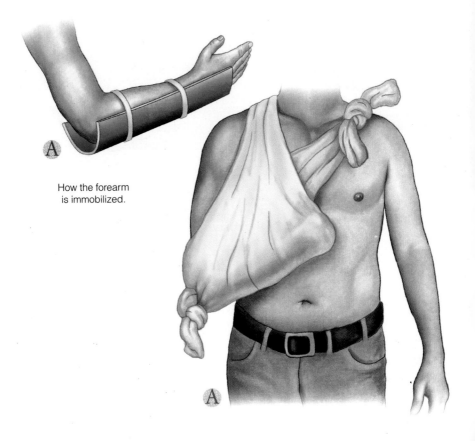

How the forearm
is immobilized.

emergency room service. On the contrary, proceed to make the immobilization of the affected arm.

Forearm fractures

- In case of not feeling the pulse in the wrist, observing limitation for the wrist, fingers or forearm movements, if the victim has numbness sensation in the hand fingers o the affected arm, the priority will be to take the victim to the closest emergency roorr service. In the opposite, carry out an immobilization of the affected arm.

HOW TO DEAL WHEN A FOREARM FRACTURE IS SUSPECTED

- Place carefully the victim's forearm at a right angle on the chest with the palm of the hand over it and the thumb pointing to the face.
- Put a cushioned immobilization that covers the lower part and the two sides of the forearm. You might use a magazine or a newspaper for doing this. The immobilization should be large enough to cover the forearm from the elbow until the wrist (avoiding the mobility of these joints). Fix the immobilization below and above the place of the fracture.
- Give stability to the immobilization by using a sling that will be tied around the neck. The sling should be placed so that the fingers (wrist) remain above the elbow level.
- Keep the victim seated while is taken to the closest emergency room service.

HOW TO MAKE AN IMMOBILIZATION OF THE COLLARBONE

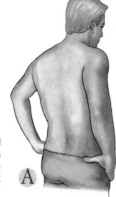

1 The injured patient is put standing as straight as possible.

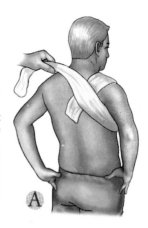

2 A wide bandage is put by starting from the midline of the back. From that place the bandage is passed over a shoulder and then under the armpit through the back toward the other shoulder.

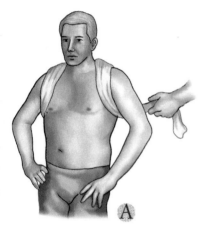

3 It is passed over the other shoulder and under the armpit…

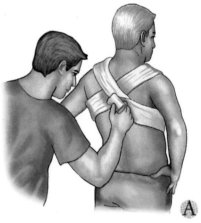

4 … until the middle of the back, in the starting point of the bandage. The bandage is placed with adhesive plaster.

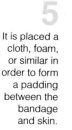
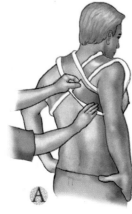

5 It is placed a cloth, foam, or similar in order to form a padding between the bandage and skin.

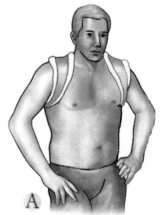

6 That is the way the bandage should be seen after is finished.

HOW TO DEAL WHEN A COLLARBONE FRACTURE IS SUSPECTED

COLLARBONE IMMOBILIZATION

- Get a large enough elastic band or bandage in order to make several turns with this around the thorax of the affected victim.
- Wrap the bandage by starting in the neck, around the victim's back diagonally, passing below the arm and then above the shoulder. Repeat this procedure by extending the bandage to the contralateral side. Repeat this procedure so that the bandage passes at least twice for each shoulder.

Collarbone fracture

- In case of a collarbone fracture is suspected, if the victim has difficulty for breathing or pain during respiration process, if it is observed an open wound in the thorax or the victim has a numbness sensation on the affected arm, contact the emergency telephone number or taken urgently the victim to the closest emergency room service. If the person does not have any of these symptoms, proceed to carry out an immobilization of the affected clavicle.

Elbow fracture

- The fractures at the elbow level have the power of causing alterations in the circulation of the affected arm. In this type of lesions is a priority to take the patient to an emergency room service in order to have a medical assessment.
- First of all, the wrist pulse should be assessed, it should also be assessed the fingers and hand movements and discard the presence of numbness or tingling in the forearm, hand and fingers. In case of having some of these symptoms, take urgently the victim to the closest emergency service.

Hand fracture

- The hand fractures are commonly more serious when the victim has difficult for moving the fingers of the affected hand, when the skin under the nails takes a bluish

HOW TO DEAL WITH AN ELBOW FRACTURE

IF AN ELBOW DEFORMITY IS OBSERVED

- Do not try to reduce or straighten out the present deformity.
- Rest forearm of the affected side on a sling, by fixing the sling to the neck of the victim.
- As much as possible, fix the affected forearm to the thorax of the victim with a towel or blanket that completely wrap both the sling and the forearm and thorax and attached it to the lower armpit of the opposite side of the lesion.

HOW TO DEAL WHEN A HAND FRACTURE IS SUSPECTED

- Bend the victim's elbow of the affected side by making an angle of 90°.
- Put a cushioned immobilization from the elbow to the victim's hand and which covers the lower part and the two sides of the limb. Make the immobilization with a clothing strip, with a tape or tie in order to keep it stable.
- As much as possible, fix the affected forearm to the victim's thorax with a towel or sheet which completely covers both the sling and the forearm and thorax and fix it to the lower armpit of the opposite site of the lesion.

HOW TO IMMOBILIZE FRACTURED LIMBS

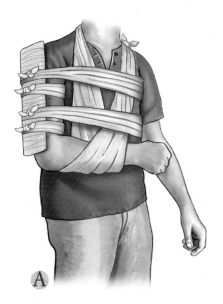

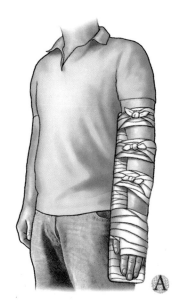

- The immobilization of the fractures is based on the splinting.
- While medical assistance arrives, some objects might be improvised to immobilize the fractured member. Woods, cardboards, newspapers, metal bars, etc. also bandages or something that substitutes for completely immobilizing the limb.
- Once the fracture has been splinted, the limb has to be placed high.
- A joint has to be immobilized above and under the injury.

- If there are not these elements, in case of having a broken arm, the fracture has to be fixed to the thorax. In case of a broken leg, it has to be immobilized to the sound leg.
- When the fracture has been immobilized, it has to be kept in the same position after the accident, keeping it at rest.
- The slings are used for different types of injuries, yet more frequently for fractures or dislocations of the arms or shoulders. In order to stabilize an injury, a piece of long and square cloth could be taken to make a triangular sling.

Something that should not be done:

- Move without care the fracture area. It should be kept the fractured area in the position that it was found.
- Do not try to realign a fractured limb. It is dangerous that might appear ruptured blood vessels with irregular sides of the fracture, something that is frequent in open fractures.
- It should not been forgotten the injury in an open fracture and be careful to avoid a possible contamination or infection of the injury.
- Do not apply ointments or use bandages after applying them because with this could be spread the risk of an allergic reaction.

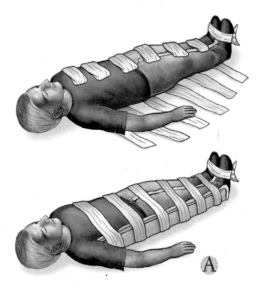

HOW TO DEAL WHEN A SHOULDER FRACTURE IS SUSPECTED

- Put the affected arm of the victim on his chest with the elbow bent a right angle.
- Put the sling and fix it to the victim's neck.
- Fix the affected arm of the victim to the body by using a towel or sheet and tying the arm under the armpit.
- Take the victim to the nearest emergency center as a priority; keep the victim seated during transfer.

HOW TO DEAL IF A KNEECAP FRACTURE IS SUSPECTED

- As much as possible, totally extend the victim's leg. However, do not do it if the victim feels much pain or it is noticeable the block sensation on the knee.
- Put a cushioned wood board or cardboard of 10 cm in width under the affected leg, in the whole leg from the hip to the ankle. Apply extra cushioned elements in the knee area and the ankle (towels, dressings, garments, etc.).
- Fix the immobilization by tying it at the ankle level, just below and above the knee and at the thigh muscle. Do not fix the immobilization above the kneecap.
- Faced the impossibility of using a wood stick or cardboard, fix the affected leg to the other leg.

coloration or when there are changes in the fingers of the affected hand sensitivity (numbness, tingling, etc). If any of these symptoms occur, as a priority, take the victim to the closest emergency service; otherwise, begin to immobilize the affected hand.

Shoulder fracture

- If a shoulder fracture is suspected, you might assess the pulse at the wrist level, in case of being unconscious or in the case of a high impact trauma, as a priority, take the victim to the closest emergency room service.

Fracture of the kneecap

- The alarm signals that suggest a complicated kneecap fracture include the loss of feeling in the leg (under the trauma level, for instance numbness, tingling, etc.), the limitation or inability to walk or for extending the whole knee, the change of skin coloration under the lesion level and the presence of an open wound (open fracture). In the presence of any of these symptoms, take urgently the victim to the nearest emergency service, otherwise, first make the immobilization of the affected leg.

Fracture of the thigh

- The lesions of fractures at the thigh muscle level might be caused by internal bleeding, which is a situation that potentially may involve the victim's life. In case of having seeing the trauma and this has a great impact, or if it is clear the presence of redness and inflammation, as a priority, take the victim to the closest emergency room service or contact the local emergency telephone number.
- Other symptoms which suggest severity or high possibility of complication related to a fracture in the thigh include the leg numbness below the trauma level, the impossibility or limitation for the extension of the leg and for walking, bluish coloration of the skin below the level lesion and the presence of an open wound. These symptoms are enough for taking the decision of transferring the victim to the nearest emergency service. Otherwise, proceed to make a thigh immobilization before taking the patient to the emergency room service.

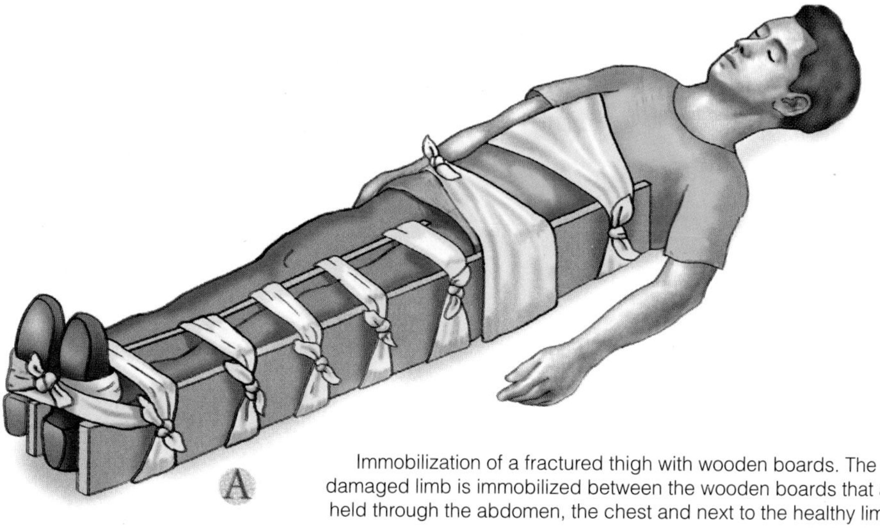

Immobilization of a fractured thigh with wooden boards. The damaged limb is immobilized between the wooden boards that are held through the abdomen, the chest and next to the healthy limb.

HOW TO DEAL WHEN A FRACTURE AT THE THIGH LEVEL IS SUSPECTED	
IF A WOODEN BOARD IS AVAILABLE FOR THE IMMOBILIZATION	IF A WOODEN BOARD IS NOT AVAILABLE FOR THE IMMOBILIZATION.
• Through a soft movement, slowly try to extend the leg. • Have at least seven strips of cloth or bandages for attaching the wooden boards. • Put two wood sticks in order to immobilize the affected thigh, the first one should be long enough to cover the distance from the armpit to the ankle. The shortest wooden board should go from the groin to the ankle. • Fix the wood sticks by tying the strips of cloth on the outside wood board (the longer of the two).	• By means of a kind movement, try to extend the leg slowly. • Provide cushioned things to put among the legs of the victim. • Fix the injured leg (fractured) to the healthy leg. The legs should be tied at the ankles level, above and below of the knee and at the thigh level. Do not fix the legs at the level of a fracture or injure.

HOW TO DEAL WHEN A LEG FRACTURE IS SUSPECTED	
WHEN THERE ARE WOODEN BOARDS TO IMMOBILIZE	WHEN THERE ARE NO BOARDS TO IMMOBILIZE
• Use at least two wooden boards, one to each side of the affected leg. As much as possible, put a third wood board in the back of the leg. The wooden boards should have a minimum length which allows immobilizing from the upper knee to much more below the ankle. • Fix the wooden boards with a cloth of strip or with bandages in at least four sites, without doing directly on the fracture.	• Gently extend the victim's leg in case of being necessary. This action could significantly reduce the pain. • Put cushioned things between the victim's legs. • Fix the injured (fractured) leg to the uninjured leg. The legs should be tied to the ankle level, above and below the knee and at the thigh level. Do not fix the legs to the injure or fracture level.

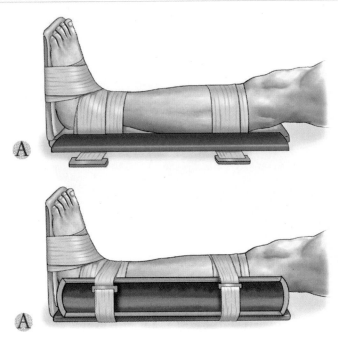

Immobilization of the leg by using wooden boards when a fracture is suspected.

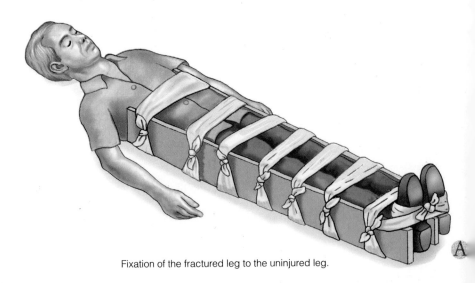

Fixation of the fractured leg to the uninjured leg.

Leg fracture

- When there is a suspicion of leg fracture and observing numbness of the leg below the trauma level, inability or limitation for extending the leg and also for walking, bluish coloration of the skin below the lesion's level and / or presence of an open injure, it has to be taken the decision of transferring the victim to the closest emergency service. Otherwise, proceed to carry out the thigh immobilization before taking the victim the emergency service.

HOW TO PREVENT MUSCLE ACHES

- Muscle aches are produced by the excessive effort of the muscles, which causes the breakage of the fibers, causing an inflammatory reaction in the affected muscle.

- Muscle aches are painful because the broken cells that are part of the damaged fibers, release substances such as calcium and potassium that are irritating and painful.

- In order to recover from muscle aches and lower the inflammation of the muscle, it will be enough to put the joint or the weak zone in a pan of water and a little of ice.

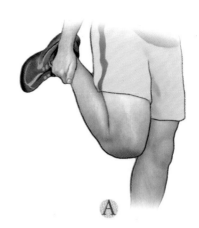

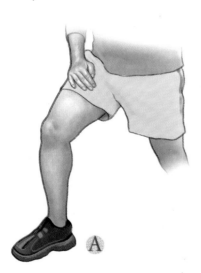

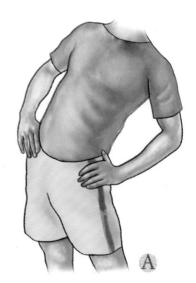

For recovering from the muscle aches, the only prevention is the regular and gradual exercise and the application of cold in the affected area.

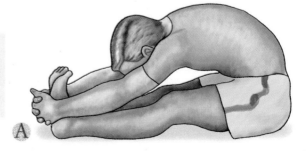

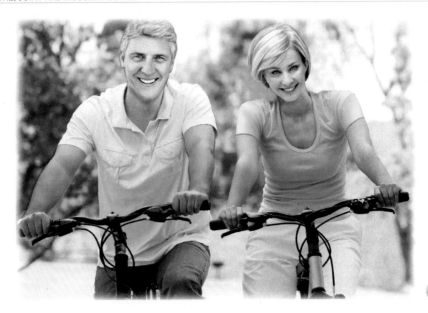

HOW TO DEAL WITH A FRACTURE OR A FRACTURE OF THE PELVIS IS SUSPECTED

- Contact the emergency telephone number or take urgently the victim to the nearest emergency room service. The fractures of the pelvis might cause severe internal bleeding, that is why the medical support and assessment has to be a priority.
- Keep the victim lying down on his back.
- The legs might be straight or flexed at the knees, anything what gives the victim less pain and greater comfort.
- Fix the legs at the level of ankles and knees, regardless of whether the knees are straight or bent.
- In case of taking the victim to the emergency room service before receiving medical support, the victim has to be placed on a rigid surface in order to reduce the complications risk. It is possible to use a portable rigid backboard, a wooden board or a door. Make sure of fixing the victim to the rigid surface with belts, bandages or strips of cloth.

Muscle strains

- Muscle strains are caused as a result of the overstraining and stretching of a particular muscle.

SYMPTOMS ASSOCIATED TO MUSCLE STRAIN

- A piercing pain in the affected area which is worse with movement.
- Inflammation of the affected zone.

HOW TO DEAL WITH A MUSCLE STRAIN

- The injured area should be resting.
- Apply ice through a towel or cold compresses to the affected area. 7-10 minutes of cold and about 30-40 minutes of resting time during the first 24 hours.
- In the next 24 hours apply compresses with warm water on the affected area.
- Elevate the affected limb above the heart level.
- Consult with the closest emergency room service in case of pain and inflammation get worse.

HOW TO PREVENT BACK ACHES

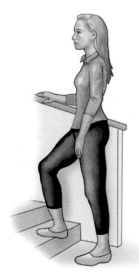

1 Standing position. When the person is standing up, the body weight has to be distributed evenly. If the person is standing for a while, the foot has to be put on a box or low stool or the rung of a ladder.

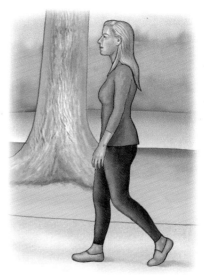

2 When walking. Keep the head up, shoulders back and raise the chest.

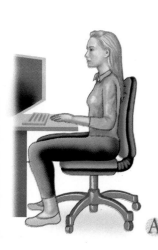

3 Seated. When the person is seated, the back has to be straight and leaned in the back of the chair, with the two feet flat on the ground or on a footrest. It is very important to avoid "being collapsed" in a chair.

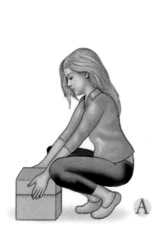
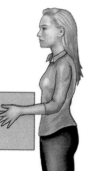

4 How to lift objects.
- The movements have to be slow and soft. Fast movements and shakes could excessively force the muscles of the back.
- Keep the body in front of the object while is lifted. Turn sideways while that object is lifted might cause a back injury.
- Keep the object near the body. Having to reach out to lift and carry an object might be harmful.

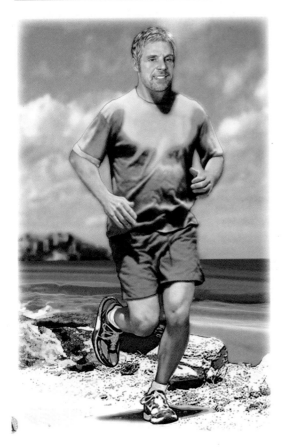

Muscle strains, muscle cramps, or sprains might occur when physical exercise with particular intensity. In order to avoid them, it is necessary to be prepared before doing that physical exercise.

HOW TO DEAL FROM A MUSCLE CRAMP

FOOT

- Move the toes toward the body.

CALF

- Stand up by leaning most of the body weight over the healthy side and massage the affected area.

BACK PART OF THE THIGH

- Lie face down and ask for a massage on the affected area of the thigh.

Muscle cramps

- The muscle cramps are commonly very painful during the nocturnal sleep, particularly in the feet, calves or in the back of the thigh. The cramps appear as a consequence of fatigue when staying at the same position for a long time or when altering the limb circulation. Local massages might be effective when stimulating the circulation.

HOW TO DEAL WITH A STRAIN

ANKLE OR KNEE STRAIN	• Apply intermittently cold compresses or ice wrapped in a towel on the affected area for 7-10 minutes and 30-40 minutes break. Do not apply warm in the first 24 hours.
	• Apply a bandage on the affected area. *(See fractures section).*
	• Keep the affected area at the heart level.
	• After the first 24 hours, apply intermittently local warm.
	• Consult a doctor in order to establish the severity of the injure.
SHOULDER, ELBOW OR WRIST STRAIN	• Use a sling on the affected limb. *(See fractures section).*
	• Apply intermittently cold compresses or ice wrapped in a towel on the affected area for 7-10 minutes and 30-40 minutes break. Do not apply warm in the first 24 hours.
	• Consult a doctor in order to establish the severity of the injure.

SYMPTOMS ASSOCIATED TO A SPRAIN

- Crack or popping or clicking sensation at the moment of the injure.
- Pain when moving the affected joint or when touching the affected area.
- Inflammation of the joint.
- Disconmfort and tenderness of the affected area.
- Blue, green or purple coloration of the affected area.

TYPES OF WOUNDS

A wound is the loss of tissue continuity, in this case the skin. There might be different wounds types:

- Sharp injuries. It is caused by sharp objects (cans, glasses, knives), that might cut muscles, tendons and nerves. The edges of the wounds are clean and lineal, the hemorrhage might be variable about the amount of blood, depending on the area of the body that has suffered a lesion.
- Puncture wound. It is produced by sharp objects (nails, needles, hooks or snake bites). These kinds of wounds are painful, in addition of having internal and external hemorrhages. The wound might be dangerous according to the deep level of the wound that reaches and the area of the body where the object penetrates (abdomen) and if there is an infection risk.
- Puncture and sharp injuries. They are caused by sharp objects (knives, daggers, screwdrivers, or a fractured bone). It is a combination of the last two kinds of injuries.
- Painful wound. It is caused by objects with jagged edges (saws). There are tissue tears and the edges are not straight or well shaped.
- Abrasive wound. It is caused by friction or rub of the skin with rough surfaces. There is a loss of the most superficial skin (epidermis), pain, type of burning that ends soon, poor hemorrhages.
- Avulsiva. It is the wound in which the tissue tears and separates from the body of the injured patient. A sharp or painful wound might become avulsiva. The bleeding is very heavy. An example of this wound might be a bite.
- A bruise wound. It is caused by blunt objects (sticks, stones, punches). There is pain and hematoma. These wounds might appear with tear of the skin, fractures and hemorrhages.
- Bruise. Closed wound caused by compression. There are internal hemorrhages that are purple.

Joint injures

Sprains

- The sprains are injuries of the ligaments which are the structures that join the bones to each other in the joints. The ligaments might be injured if they are completely strained or broken when a joint exceeds the range of normal motion, mainly through sprains.

SKIN INJURES AND SUPERFICIAL TRAUMAS

SKIN INJURES AND SUPERFICIAL TRAUMAS

Superficial hitting

- Superficial hits or bruises are the most common injuries. These types of injuries appear after a hit or fall as a result of the blood vessels break. The coloration changes

SYMPTOMS ASSOCIATED TO SUPERFICIAL HITS

- Pain.
- Change of the initial coloration to bluish or red tones.
- Change of the coloration to green tones.
- A bump associated to the hematoma formation
- The area has a yellowish coloration and after that brown, before disappearing completely the coloration change.

HOW TO DEAL WITH A SUPERFICIAL HITTING

- As a priority, apply cold compresses or an ice bag on the affected area; do not apply directly the ice on the skin because it could be burnt by the cold. The ice might be applied by using a towel or a garment. Local cold reduces inflammation and bleeding which are related to the trauma.
- If the hitting is on a limb (arm, leg), elevate it above the heart level in order to reduce blood flow. Do not apply tourniquets.
- After the first 24 or 48 hours of the trauma, apply local wet heat in a compress (towel, dressing, garment which are wet with hot water). The local warm stimulates the blood circulation to the affected area in order to help healing.
- If the victim had a high impact hitting or if the pain does not stop and the inflammation progresses, as a priority, consult with a doctor in order to discard the presence of fractures or greater severe injuries.

WHAT TO DO IN CASE OF BUMPS

- First of all, it should be tried to reduce the pain. With this small device will be applied an ice pack (never apply ice directly to the skin) on the affected zone for about 15 minutes.
- It will be tried to keep immobilized the affected area.
- In case of having a wound, it should be washed with running water and do not apply creams or ointments.
- If there are no wounds an anti inflammatory or analgesic ointment should be applied.
- If the contusion is severe and it is on the leg it should be kept high for some hours.
- The affected area should not be strongly massaged or rubbed.
- Do not empty the hematomas or prick the wound.
- It is possible to take paracetamol or ibuprofen for the pain, although aspirins are not recommended because they could increase the size of the hematoma.
- If the pain continues and the injured limb cannot be moved, you should go to a health center.

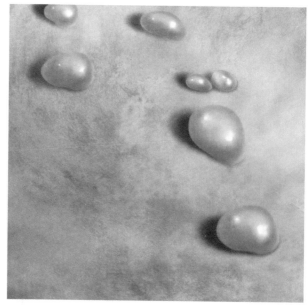

The blisters are lesions caused by an irregular elevation of the round or oval shape epidermis. They might appear as a vesicle with fine walls which is localized on the skin and mucous. At the beginning contains a clear and serous liquid that later on might contain blood and/or pus. They might vary in size, from 1cm of diameter to 10cm.

and the associated inflammation are the consequence of the blood release from the blood vessels to the superficial tissues; they are changing as the hit is suffering the normal healing process.

HOW TO DEAL WITH BLISTERS

• If the blister is small, it will not get further irritation.	• Apply a little of petroleum jelly (vaseline) and cover the blister with a sterile gauze. The liquid inside the blister will be reabsorbed by itself.
• If the blister breaks and the subcutaneous tissues are exposed.	• Wash carefully the blister with water and soap. Do not apply alcohol or other medicines, or home remedies. • Apply the vaseline on the blister and cover it with sterile gauze.
• If the blister is big and is high the probability of breaking up the blister because of the daily activities.	• As much as possible, look for medical attention for treating the blister. • If it is not possible to get medical attention: • Wash carefully the blister area with water and soap. • Sterilize a needle by putting it on the fire. • Press the lower side of the blister, by softly pressing the blister helping to remove the liquid inside it. • Wash again with water and soap, apply a little of vaseline and cover with a sterile gauze. • Periodically assess the presence of infection signals such as temperature increase of the area to the palpation area, redness, hardening or pus production. Look for medical attention in case of observing these symptoms.

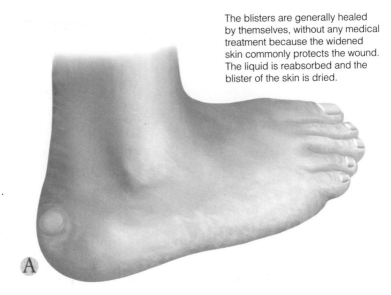

The blisters are generally healed by themselves, without any medical treatment because the widened skin commonly protects the wound. The liquid is reabsorbed and the blister of the skin is dried.

Blisters

- Blisters are commonly cause by clothing, shoes or apparel which produce repetitive rubber with the skin. The best way of treating blisters is by healing by themselves, helping the hydration and lubrication of the affected area.

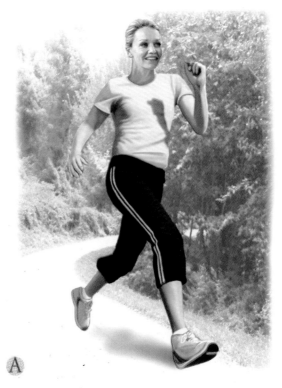

Long walks, especially if they are in the mountain, if there are not appropriate measures, particularly about the worn shoes, might have the risk of causing blisters which are always annoying and painful.

RESPIRATORY EMERGENCIES

Asthma attacks

- Asthma is a medical condition which appears as a result of the progressive narrowing (sometimes sudden, asthma attacks) of the airways as a result of the exposure of some substances or environmental conditions, producing breathing difficulty, particularly exhaling (expel the air).

- Generally, an asthma attack is the consequence of the victim's exposure to a substance to which the person became allergic. Other factors that might cause an asthma attack are the infections (common flu, tonsillitis, sinusitis, bronchitis, etc.), the exercise, cold environments or sudden temperature changes, inhaled irritant in the environment or even emotional factors may cause an asthma attack.

- Asthmatic people that regularly exercise or start an exercise routine, should keep the inhaler at hand, especially those people who practice swimming because the exercise favors the sudden temperature and humidity changes associated to swimming, might cause asthmatic attacks.

CHARACTERISTICS SYMPTOMS OF AN ASTHMA CRISIS

- Breathing difficulty (expel the air), it is possible to hear a whistle blowing or buzzing which is similar to the air passage through a tube.
- Keep seated in order to improve or facilitate breathing, increase of the symptoms when lying down or standing up.
- Anxiety, tension, fear.
- Coughing.
- Sweating on the forehead.
- Vomitting.
- Fever.
- Bluish coloration of the skin as a consequence of the decreased blood oxygen levels.
- Suffocating sensation.

STEPS TO FOLLOW FROM AN INITIAL EPISODE OF ASTHMA (ASTHMA IS SUSPECTED)

- Look for medical attention as a priority.
- Report with details the observed events during the episode.
- In case of not being possible to contact a doctor, take the victim to the nearest emergency center.
- Stay with the victim and keep him calm in order to observe any change and to reduce the possibility of emotional stress.
- Keep the victim in a seated position, do not lay the patient.

STEPS TO FOLLOW FROM AN ASTHMA EPISOSE IN A PERSON WHO HAS HAD PREVIOUS EPISODES

- Give the prescribed medicines according to the doctor's recommendations (if you know them) or according to the medicine bottle.
- Do not give the victim anything else without medical approval.
- Consult and inform to the treating physician the situation.
- In case of persisting the symptoms or being related with some of the next conditions, look for medical attention as a matter of priority:
  - If there is no improvement despite of giving the medication properly.
  - Difficulty for inhaling or inability to exhale (breathing is not normally heard).
  - Inability for speaking or coughing.
  - Increase or appearance of a bluish skin color, particularly around the mouth or in the nail bed.
  - Increase of the pulse which is more than 120 beats per minute.
  - Increase of the respiration rate to more than 30 heart beats per minute.
  - Increase of the anxiety, related sweating.
  - Persistent and uncontrolled coughing.
  - Nasal flaring in children.
  - Grunting or moaning sound in children.
  - Inability to breathe when lying down.

SIGNS OF RESPIRATORY FAILURE

- If the victim elevates the shoulders or extends the chin in his effort for breathing and take air to the lungs, contact the emergency telephone number or take the victim to the nearest emergency room service as a priority. These signs precede the respiratory failure and the victim is about to lose the conscious state.

CROUP

- Croup refers to the group of respiratory symptoms associated to several respiratory conditions which appear in children younger than 3 years old. Croup is caused for

HOW TO ACT FROM A CROUP EPISODE

- Keep calm and avoid that the child is scared.
- Do not put any object in the kid's mouth, this practice does not improve the respiratory pattern and it might favor the obstruction of the airway.
- Use a vaporizer in the child's bedroom in order to improve the respiratory pattern. One alternative option is to be seated with the child in the bathroom with the door closed and with the shower running in warm water to promote the steam produced by the water. Do not put the child under the shower running. Stay inside the bathroom for 20 or 30 minutes.
- Contact the local telephone emergency number or take the child to closest emergency service if the symptoms persist or if it is observed any of the next situations:
  - The conditions worsen despite of the child being awake.
  - Progressive difficulty for breathing.
  - Noisy breathing when inhaling despite of the child being calm
  - Bluish coloration of the skin and lips.
  - Fever.
  - Agitation, tiredness or inability for doing common activities.
  - Decreased muscle tone.

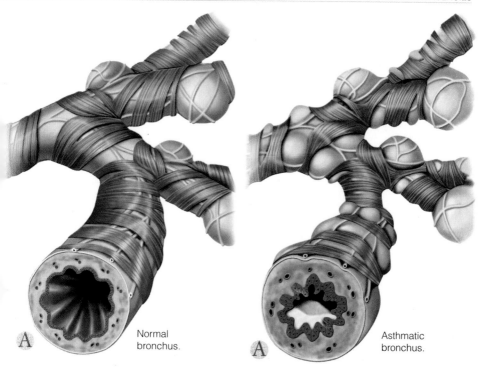

Normal bronchus.

Asthmatic bronchus.

The bronchial asthma is a respiratory disease characterized by the chronic inflammation of the air way (bronchi), which causes recurrent episodes of air lack sensation (dyspnea), chest feels wheezy with breathing (wheeze), cough and chest tight.

SYMPTOMS ASSOCIATED TO THE CROUP

- Difficulty breathing, especially difficulty for taking the air.
- Stridor when inhaling (noisy breathing).
- Hoarseness.
- Barking cough.
- Bluish coloration of the skin and lips.
- Fatigue, trouble sleeping.

viral or bacterial infections and as a consequence of allergic reactions. It commonly appears in spring, winter and rain seasons.
- Croup attacks are mainly observed in the nights when the child has gone to sleep in a time which is related with a cold or respiratory virus. When croup shows its symptoms during the day, it commonly gets worse at night.

EPIGLOTTITIS SYMPTOMS

- Difficulty for swallowing or passing foods and liquids.
- Increased salivation and drooling.
- Dysphonia, changes of the characteristics of the voice, loss voice.
- Fever
- The child has a seated position with the open mouth and the protrude jaw trying to increase the air flow and keep open the airway.

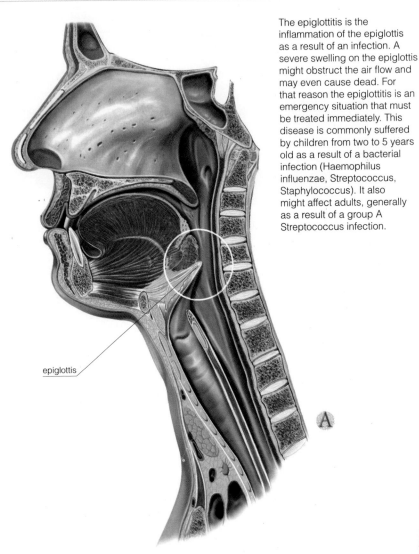

The epiglottitis is the inflammation of the epiglottis as a result of an infection. A severe swelling on the epiglottis might obstruct the air flow and may even cause dead. For that reason the epiglottitis is an emergency situation that must be treated immediately. This disease is commonly suffered by children from two to 5 years old as a result of a bacterial infection (Haemophilus influenzae, Streptococcus, Staphylococcus). It also might affect adults, generally as a result of a group A Streptococcus infection.

epiglottis

A

Epiglottitis

- The epiglottitis is a serious medical condition that might threaten the affected person's life. This appears when the epiglottis (structure of the cartilage that closes the trachea when swallowing) suffers and infection, inflammation or swelling, blocking partially the airway. The epiglottitis is mainly observed in children between 2 and 7 years old, after having had flu, sore throat and sore hoarseness episodes.

HOW TO DEAL WITH A SUSPECTED EPIGLOTTITIS EPISODE

- Contact the local telephone number for emergencies or take urgently the child to the nearest emergency room service keeping the kid always seated.
- Do not put any object in the child's mouth, this procedure does not improve the respiratory pattern and might promote the obstruction of the airway.
- Do not make the child agitated; avoid the effort and physical activity. Keep calm and keep the child calm.

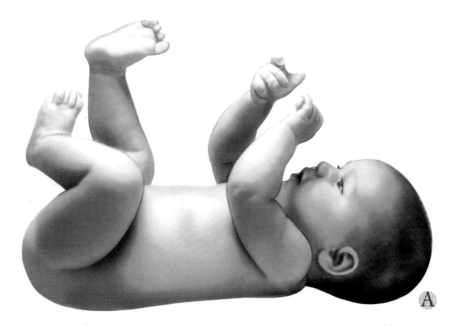

Sudden infant death syndrome is the sudden and unexpected dead of a child younger than one year old. The cause is unknown, however some researchers think that is cause by problems of the baby for waking up or the inability of the baby's body to detect the accumulation of the carbon dioxide on the blood.

HOW TO DEAL WITH A SUDDEN INFANT DEATH SYNDROME

- Contact your local emergency telephone number.
- Try to restore breathing and circulation. (See chapter about cardiopulmonary resuscitation).

HOW TO PREVENT SUDDEN INFANT DEATH SYNDROME

- Always place the baby on his or her back.
- Make sure that the mattress is firm and flat.
- Never allow that the baby sleep on a puff, water bed or other piece of furniture with a soft surface.
- Do not allow that the child sleeps with stuffed, soft toys, pillows or comforters.
- Do not allow the baby build up heat to dangerous levels; do not exceed clothes or blankets for doing that the child sleeps.
- Do not use plastic blankets.
- Do not allow smoking near the area where children sleep.

Sudden infant death syndrome

- The sudden infant death syndrome is the death of a baby apparently healthy younger than one year old, more frequent at 6 months without a clear or apparent cause.

BURNS

- The main objective from a burn is to relieve the associated pain as a matter of priority. Complementary it is important to act in order to reduce risk infections and prevent or treat complications as a systemic shock. The initial treatment of a burn by the person who provides first aid lies in reducing the temperature on the burnt area, reducing the risk of complications on the affected tissues under the influence of heat.

- The burns caused by sun, fires (flames) or by hot substances are qualified according to the damage caused; the first degree burns are less severe, second degree are intermediate and third degree are the most severe ones.

First degree-burns

- First degree-burns are characterized by only superficial tissue damage (the most external layers of the skin). Sun burns, by the direct contact but for a short-term with objects or hot substances or steam burns are the ones that most frequently produce first degree-burns. This kind of burns are completely healed after 7 or 10 days.

FIRST DEGREE-BURNS

- The first degree burns are those that affect the epidermis, or superficial CAPA of the skin. That skin reds and dries, it hurts, causes a burning sensation and it becomes slightly inflamed.

- If the burn has not affected big surfaces of the hands, feet, face or groins, the next cares could be followed:

  - Apply compresses of cold and wet wipes or submerge the affected part in clean cold water, nevertheless, no so much.

  - It is also recommended to run clean water on the burn. Keep the burn under the running water, at least, for about five minutes or until pain is mitigated.

  - In the case of a child, he should be calmed and told that this problem does not need much attention.

  - After the burn has been under running water, it will be covered with a non adhesive sterile bandage, or with a towel or a clean piece of clothing.

  - It is important to protect the burn from pressures or rubs.

  - Do not apply ointments, because they might cause infection. When the skin is cold, it could be applied a moisturizing lotion.

  - Some pain relieve medicines might be applied (paracetamol, aspirin, ibuprofen) without medical prescription, in order to relieve the pain and reduce inflammation.

  - The first degree burns are commonly healed without any treatment. However, if it is a first degree burn that covers a big area of the body, or if the victim is a child or an elderly, it will be needed to go to the medical emergency.

  - It should be verified that the injured has received the anti tetanus vaccine.

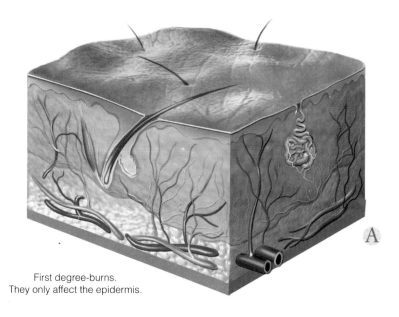

First degree-burns.
They only affect the epidermis.

SYMPTOMS ASSOCIATED TO FIRST DEGREE-BURNS

- Pain.
- Redness around the affected area.
- Mild swelling.
- Intact skin, it is not observed the presence of blisters.

HOW TO ACT TO A FIRST DEGREE-BURNS

- Immediately after a burn is presented, the affected area must be put under cold running water or apply a compress with cold water until pain lessens.
- Cover the burn with a clean or sterile bandage. Do not apply any type of fatty substance into the wound. Do not apply any medicine neither home remedies on the burn without a doctor's authorization.

Second degree-burns

- Burns which induce damage on deep layers of the skin are called second degree-burns. Prolonged exposure to the sun, hot liquids and gasoline flames or other fuels, are the principal causes of this type of burn. Healing can take about 3 weeks.

ASSOCIATED SYMPTOMS TO A SECOND DEGREE-BURNS

- Evident redness, also is possible to observe patches or lines of different tone on the affected area.
- Presence of blisters.
- Inflammation which can last more than 2 weeks.
- Wet look or viscosity of the area.
- Pain.

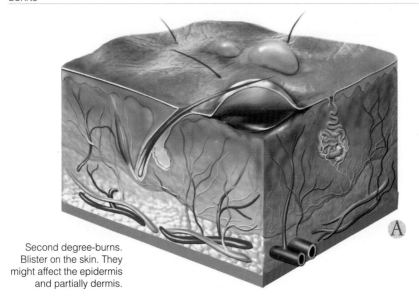

Second degree-burns.
Blister on the skin. They
might affect the epidermis
and partially dermis.

SECOND DEGREE-BURNS

- The second degree burns are those which affect the epidermis in its bottom layer, or dermis. The skin gets red, hurts, blisters appear, discharges pus and the skin starts to shed.
- In the case of second degree burns, the next advices should be followed:
  - Apply cold compresses or wipes, or submerge the affected part in clean water, it is important not to leave for a long time.
  - It is also useful to put the burn under cold water. Continue until the pain is relieved or at least for at least for about minutes.
  - Once the burns have been for a while under running water, they will be covered with a adhesive sterile bandage or with a towel or clean piece of cloth.
  - Do not touch the blisters.
  - Do not apply ointments, because they could cause infection.
  - If the child is scared, place lying down with the feet elevated.
  - If the burn area is more than 5 cm of diameter, it is necessary to go to the medical center.

HOW TO DEAL WITH A SECOND DEGREE-BURNS

- Introduce the affected area in cold water without ice. Alternatively may apply cold compresses on the affected area. Any available beverage and which is found to a lower temperature of the environment may be dumped on the burn. Do this procedure until pain decreases or relieves completely. The main objective is to reduce the temperature of the affected area to reduce the likelihood of tissue damage. Do not apply ice, since it may induce a burn by cold in a tissue already injured by heat.
- Dry the affected area with a clean and dry towel or other clothing.
- Remove any accessory present in the affected area (jewelry, handles, rings, earrings, etc.)
- Cover the affected area with a bandage or soft and clean clothing to prevent associated infections. For any reason try to break blisters or apply medicines, creams, oils or other home remedies on the affected area.
- In case that the burn is on a limb, raise it above heart level in order to reduce the blood flow and the associated inflammation.
- Look for medical assistance as a matter of priority. Assess the presence of burns around the mouth and nose, if you observe burning hair on these areas tell the doctor in order to discard breathing complications associated to toxic inhalations and smoke.

SKIN STRUCTURE

tactile corpuscle of Vater-Pacini
nerve
arteriole
venule
subcutaneous adipose tissue
tactile corpuscle of Krause
tactile corpuscle of Ruffini
sensory nerve
tactile corpuscle of Meissner
sebaceous gland
capillary network of hair root
nervous plexus of root hair
sweat gland
receptor Merkel cell
sweat gland (eccrine)
involved duct
arrector of hair
sweat pore
hair follicle
hair root
hair stem
dermis papillae
basal cell layer
stratum spinosum
epidermis
granular layer
stratum lucidum
stratum corneum
spiral duct
papillary region
reticular region
epidermis
dermis
hypodermis

67

ASSOCIATED SYMPTOMS TO A THIRD DEGREE-BURNS

- White or corrugated skin on the affected area.
- Evident damage of skin.
- Pain is not so intense since nervous ends generally look affected.

THIRD DEGREE-BURNS

- The third degree burns are extended to the deep tissues, making the skin that becomes of colors that might vary between White, Brown, yellow and even black, and the sensitivity is lost due to the destruction of the nerve endings. The dry skin has a refined aspect. It is also observed swelling of the tissues.
- In case of having third degree burns, the next advices should be followed:
  - If there is an extended area, they might be life threatening endangered the victim's life. It means that these lesions require immediate medical assistance.
  - In the emergency room, the health personnel will make sure that the burn might breathe appropriately, with this will be proved that other injuries do not endangered the burn patient's life and a treatment will be started in order to restore loss liquids and avoid infections.

Third degree-burns

- The burns that wholly destroy the entire skin layer are called third degree burns. Fire, the prolonged contact with objects or hot substances and electrical burns are the main causes of third degree burns.

HOW TO DEAL WITH A THIRD DEGREE-BURNS

- If victim shows flames (fire) in some place of his/her corporal surface, control the fire completely with a sufficiently thick sheet or clothing.
- Try to contact the local number of emergencies or the victim must be taken to the nearest emergency service, as a matter of priority.
- Verify frequently the breathing pattern of the victim, keeps the air way open. Breathing difficulty is a frequent symptom of third degree-burns, especially in facial which compromise nose or mouth or has implied smoking inhalation.
- Apply cold clothing or a cold compress on the affected area by the burn. Do not apply ice.
- Cover the burn with clean clothing, preferably made of cotton which does not release speckles or feathers.
- In case that the burn is on a limb, raise it above heart level in order to reduce the blood flow and the associated inflammation.
- Do not allow the victim to walk, particularly in the low limbs burns.
- If the burn was on the face or neck, provides support to these areas with a pillow to keep upright neck.
- Monitor and assess shock presence, shown by a serious difficulty for breathing or decreasing alertness or pulse. If you suspect shock presence follow the next instructions:
  - Keeps the victim lying down unless burns are presented on the face or neck.
  - Elevate the victim's legs 20-25 cm, placing a bench under his/her heels, unless victim is unconscious or shows significant injuries on the face, neck or chin.
  - If the is found unconscious or shows injuries on the face level, neck or chin arrange her/him sideways with the neck extended.
  - Allow the victim to keep his/her stable body temperature, covering her/him with a blanket; place a sheet under the victim if he/she is found directly in contact with the floor.
  - Do not give liquids or any food.
  - Keep calm and keep the victim calm.

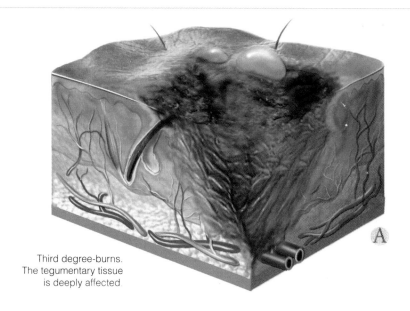

Third degree-burns.
The tegumentary tissue
is deeply affected.

CHEMICAL BURNS

- They are caused by chemical substances and they might be very dangerous because they penetrate the skin, damaging the muscles, bones, nerves, tendons and other important tissues.

- These types of burns cause one of the most complex emergencies to handle, for both the action mechanisms of the different chemical products and for the great number of product that there are in several aspects of the life. It is calculated that in the current society there are more than 25.000 of agricultural, industrial or domestic use which may cause burns.

- Most of the chemical burns are produced accidentally and most of them are mild and they could be cased at home. However, it should not be forgotten the high number of aggressions which are produced by this type of those products.

- The prevention is very important in this type of burns. Especially in the work, it is necessary to pay attention to the respect about security measures that are in place. Never forget that manipulating this type of products is dangerous.

- The management of chemical burns should be made by specialized personnel.

- In case of having a chemical burn, the next steps should be followed:
  - Check that the burn cause has been eliminated. For that will be put the burn under running water for at least 20 minutes to make sure the disappearance of the chemical substance that has caused that burn.
  - Remove clothing and beads which are contaminated by the substance that caused the burn.
  - Cover the burn area with dry sterile gauze or with a clean cloth.
  - Wash again the burn area during several minutes more if the affected individual notices that the burn sensation is intensified after the first wash.
  - Minor burns generally heal without any additional treatment.
  - It will be needed to look for medical attention if:
    - If the substance burned the external layer of the skin in the whole thickness and the resulting burn has an area more than 5-7 cm of diameter.
    - If the chemical burn affected hands, feet, face, groin, buttocks or a big joint.
    - Remove all the clothes of the burn victim and wash him with abundant water until the chemical substance has totally been eliminated.
    - Do not stop pouring clean and cold water on the burn.
    - Take immediately the injured to the nearest emergency center, or for an ambulance which might be enabled for the intensive care unit.

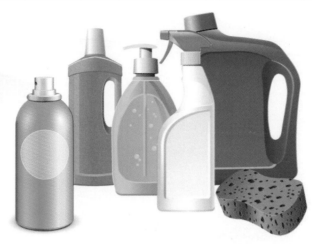

It is believed that there are currently more than 25.000 products in the world market, for domestic, agricultural and industrial use that are capable of causing different types of burns.

HOW TO DEAL WITH A CHEMICAL BURN SUSPICION

- Thoroughly wash the affected area or which entered in contact with the chemical substance with running water during at least 5 continuous minutes. The amount and flow speed of water are essential to reduce exposure of the substance and reduce the probability of tissue damage.
- Continue the wash of the affected area while you remove clothing which may have entered in contact with the chemical substance.
- As far as possible, get the chemical substance package which caused the burn, looking for the instructions on the label for a burn manage or exposure to the substance.
- Apply a cold clothing or a cool compress on the affected area by the burn. Do not apply ice.
- Cover the burn with clean clothing, preferably made of cotton which does not release speckles or feathers.
- For any reason apply medicines, creams, oils or other home remedies on the affected area.
- Look for the emergency room service, transfer the victim to the nearest emergency service.

WHAT TO DO IN ORDER TO PREVENT BURNS

- As soon as possible, put protection around the objects that are hot.
- Select and use objects which have insulating elements (handles, side-handles, etc), taking care that they in a good state.
- Use gloves or working gloves for moving hot objects or manipulating inside a heated oven.
- Avoid splashes, using silverware or lifts, while foods are cooked.
- Use the burners placed in the back, far away of the person who handles them.
- Serve the food warm.
- Keep away children in their arms while hot liquids are manipulated or they are cooked.
- Keep away children from the kitchen and the ironing room.
- Keep out of reach of children the hot objects or with living flame.
- Avoid that children play with matches, lighters, etc.
- Handle with much care bangers, flash bangers and cartridges and keep out of reach of children.
- Do not put containers with water on the stoves or the heater.
- Leave the iron on a high furniture, closed and with rolled wire.
- Keep plugs covered with furniture.
- Keep wire and electric appliances in a good state.
- Avoid the use of extension cords and overload wall outlets.
- Hide wires on the corners or under the furniture.

CALCULATION OF BODILY SURFACE

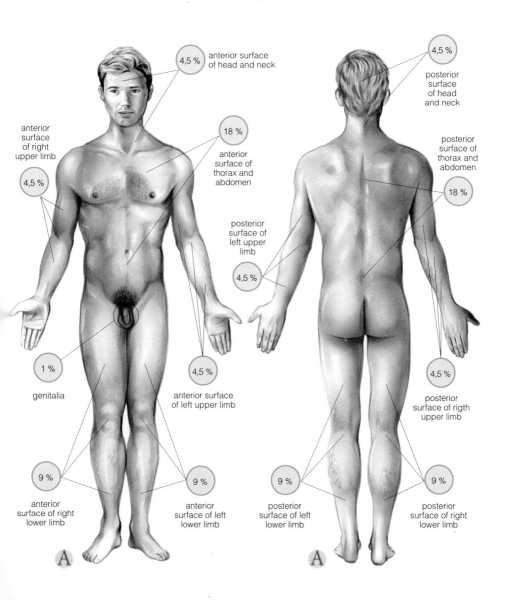

anterior surface of head and neck — 4,5 %

posterior surface of head and neck — 4,5 %

anterior surface of right upper limb — 4,5 %

anterior surface of thorax and abdomen — 18 %

posterior surface of thorax and abdomen — 18 %

posterior surface of left upper limb — 4,5 %

genitalia — 1 %

anterior surface of left upper limb — 4,5 %

posterior surface of rigth upper limb — 4,5 %

anterior surface of right lower limb — 9 %

anterior surface of left lower limb — 9 %

posterior surface of left lower limb — 9 %

posterior surface of right lower limb — 9 %

CALCULATION OF BODILY SURFACE

The calculation of bodily surface is complex because the human body has many prominences, concavities, crannies and several shapes. In certain occasions, especially when burns are produced, it is said about the percentage of the affected area. In order to establish this calculation, it is often used as a method the so called nine formula, slang that has been applied because adopts the number 9 as the base. Thus in adults, the head represents 4.5%, each upper limb is the equivalent of 4.5%, the anterior and posterior parts of the trunk are calculated each one as 18 percent, and it is also calculated in 9% each lower limp, and the remaining 1% for the genitalia.

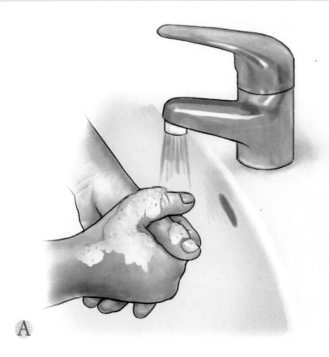

A

The first thing to do with a chemical burn is to put the burn area under running water for a long time in order to remove the causative of that burn.

GENERAL TREATMENT OF THE BURNS

- Calm down the victim and his or her relatives.
- Assess the type of burn and its severity
- Carefully remove rings, watch, bracelets, belt or tight clothing that press the injured area, before this starts to swell.
- Do not break the blisters in order to avoid infections and traumas.
- Cool down the burn area during several minutes. Apply physiological saline solution or cold water (no ice water) on the injury.
- Do not use ice to cool down the burn area, do not apply cream or ointments because they might interfere or delay the medical treatment.
- Cover the burn area with a clean dressing or moist cloth with physiological saline solution or cold clean water and hold the affected area with a bandage in order to avoid the injury contamination with pathogen germs.
- Do not press the burn
- If the burn is in hands and feet, put gauze between the fingers and toes before putting the bandage.
- If there are burns in the face or neck, put a pillow or cushion under the shoulders and control vital signs. Cover the burns of the face with sterile gauze or clean cloth, open holes for eyes, nose and mouth.
- Take the victim to a health center.

Chemical burns

- Chemical burns are presented when the victim's skin enters in contact with any chemical substance which is able to induce damage of the tissue when enter in direct contact with the skin.

INTOXICATIONS

Poisoning

- Poisonings are situations with high risk to compromise the affected individual life. In the presence of an individual who has taken poison, get in contact immediately with the emergency local number to be assisted in the attention procedure to the affected person. As far as possible have in hand the following information:
  - Individual concerned age.
  - Kind of poison.
  - Amount swallowed.
  - When was the intake.
  - Information about if individual has been vomiting.
  - How far/long is the nearest emergency room.
- The treatment and medical assistance for a poisoned individual is an emergency, medical assistance must be given as soon as possible and it must include:
  - Assessment by specialized professionals
  - Dilution of poison with milk or water. Do not give any juice.

HOW TO DEAL WITH THE INTAKE OF A POISON

IF THE VICTIM DOES NOT BREATH

- Get in contact with the local emergency number to request urgent medical assistance.
- Keep the airway opens, restore breathing and circulation if necessary
- Bring the poison container or any material as vomiting to the hospital.

IF VICTIM IS UNCONSCIOUS OR HAS CONVULSIONS

- Get in touch with emergency local number to request urgent medical attention.
- Keep the airways open; restore breathing and circulation if necessary.
- To liberate tight-fitting clothing, especially around neck, do not induce vomiting; do not give liquids or food to the victim. If individual is vomiting by his/her own, place him/her sideways to avoid that aspire the vomiting.
- Bring the poison container or any vomiting material to the hospital.

IF VICTIM IS CONSCIOUS

- Get in contact with the emergency phone number to require urgent medical assistance, without losing the sight or neglect the affected individual.
- Bring the poison container or any vomiting material to the hospital.

WHAT TO DO WITH A CAUSTIC INTOXICATION

The word caustic is applied to very aggressive substances which destroy the tissues by contact and might cause the death in a few hours or affect a person for a lifetime.

Its importance is because the most frequent caustics used are part of the majority of the products that are used in the household cleaning: detergents, deoxidants, bleaches, etc) and industrial products.

- General rules:
  - Never should be administered alkaline substances (sodium bicarbonate) in intoxications caused by acids because the union of both substances gives place to the formation of abundant gases that will ease vomiting or even might produce gastric explosion.
  - In the intoxication by alkalis, it always has to be dissolved the toxic with drinking liquids.
  - Only should be neutralized the substance in the first 10 to 15 minutes.
  - The milk might cause vomiting because of the gastric intolerance.
  - Transfer immediately the injured to the hospital.
- Rules in case of acids ingestion:
  - Do not induce vomiting to the patient.
  - Neutralize the acid with alkaline substances such as common milk or abundant water.
  - In the case of strong acids, it will be done a neutralization of chemical type, giving to the injured person a glass of magnesia.
  - Relieve the pain.
- Rules in case of alkalis ingestion:
  - The most ingested substance is the bleach.
  - Do not provoke vomiting.
  - Neutralize the alkalis with acetic acid, vinegar solution (100 cc in a liter of sugar), lemon juice, or milk solution or albumin water (4 whites of egg in a liter of water).
  - Relieve the pain.

- Extract the poison from individual. Do not induce vomiting; this maneuver only could be done if necessary by specialized professionals.

Do not induce vomiting by any reason to the following conditions:

- Individual is unconscious.
- It is unknown the type of taken poison.

WHAT TO DO WITH A POISONING THROUGH DIGESTIVE TRACT

- It is very important that the digestive system does not absorb the toxic, for this, the best method will be to produce vomiting.
- The most common method to provoke vomiting is to insert the finger in the mouth as deep as possible.
- Another method to provoke vomiting is to offer salt water, coffee, salt to the injured.
- If these methods do not work, it is possible to go to the pharmacy in order to get syrup of ipecac and drink 30 ml dissolved In 250 ml of water.
- Take the patient to the emergency room.
- It must not be produced vomiting in the next cases:
  - If it is observed burns in lips and mouth.
  - If the breathing is of kerosene, gasoline or derivatives.
  - If there are clues of having ingested caustic products or turpentine.
  - If the label of the ingested product indicates that.
  - If the injured is unconscious or has convulsions.
  - After two hours of having ingested the toxic.

INTOXICATION BY MEDICINES

Stimulants, depressants or disturbings of the central nervous system activity

- These types of medicines are sedative, anxiolytic, tranquilizer or hypnotic type.
- The symptoms will be different, depending on the effects and ingested dose, nevertheless the symptoms will be the next:
  - The injured has an unclear speaking, the person is barely understood.
  - His movements are not coordinated, if the person is given a glass with water has trouble to take it or drop it. The victim is not able to walk in a straight line and falls down easily.
  - His breathing is slowed down.
  - The pupils are smaller than normal and if they are illuminated, they do not react.
- In this type of intoxications it is necessary to follow the next steps:
  - Talk to the individual in order to avoid falling asleep.
  - Put the injured in a place where there is no danger to avoid falling in the stairs, cutting with knives, burning with cigarettes, etc.
  - Be next to the injured, and do not leave the victim at any moment.
  - Take the injured to the emergency room.

Non stimulants, depressants or disturbings of the central nervous system activity

- In this case the symptoms are different, depending the effects and dose of the medicine ingested:
  - Because the intoxication is oral, it is possible to have nausea, vomiting and diarrhea.
  - Abdomen pain.
  - Headache, vertigo, convulsions, cardio pulmonary arrest.
- In this type of intoxications is necessary:
  - Call to the emergency service center for moving immediately the injured.
  - If the intoxicated is conscious, try to make the victim to vomit, if there has been less that an hour after having ingested the medicine.
  - Look for the box of the taken medication and transfer the victim to the emergency room for being assessed by the medical personnel.
  - If the intoxicated has been vomiting, take a sample of that and carry to the emergency room.

Paracetamol

- The paracetamol is an analgesic and antipyretic, in other words, a drug that helps to reduce pain and fever. Is one of the most used medicines in children and adults and it has to be taken into account in the emergency room by intoxications. Currently its toxicity is an important cause of mortality caused by intoxications in many countries.
- When it is administered in the therapeutic dose advised by the physician, generally is well tolerated, sure and lack of toxic effects. However, when the drug exceeds five or six times the normal dose, it is produced an intoxication which has several stages:
  - It is important to remember that the symptoms that have this type of intoxication do not immediately appear, they are mild and do not warn about the severity of the symptoms that will appear later on, which are very severe or they even could cause death.
  - In the stage I, which occurs during the first 24 hours, might be produced nausea, vomiting and drowsiness, but in some intoxicated these symptoms do not appear.
  - In the stage II, which occurs between 24 and 72 hours, it could start to appear pain in the right side of the body, where the liver is located. Some intoxicated might have problems to urinate.
  - In the stage III, which occurs between 72 and 96 hours, the intoxicated might have jaundice, in other words, the skin becomes yellowish due to the damage that is caused by the paracetamol into the liver. About a quarter and half of the injured patients might present renal insufficiency.
  - In the stage IV, which occur between the fourth and the two weeks after taking paracetamol, the intoxicated that are able to survive, start to recover slowly. If it is treated in time, hepatic lesions do not leave chronic consequences.
- Treatment aims to reduce or limit the pass of the medicine to the bloodstream, which could be achieved by inducing vomiting, while medical support is received. In the hospital will be done a stomach

washing and will be used a specific antidote that if it is correctly administered, it will achieve its effect. The most recommended is to go urgently to the nearest hospital.

- In order to prevent intoxications caused by paracetamol is necessary:
  - Unfortunately, most of the cases of intoxication with paracetamol are presented in children who swallow it by accident. That is why is insisted in keeping out of the reach of children and under lock and key.
  - In the case of adult, it should be reminded that self medication is dangerous. It is necessary to consult the physician or the pharmacist before taking any medicine.

MEASURES TO PREVENT INTOXICATIONS

- Do not store medicines in a place where children can reach them.
- Do not mix medication with alcohol.
- Do not take medications with bottles without a label or if this is not legible.
- Store medications in places well ventilated.
- Do not mix household cleaning without checking the label, above all in case that the bleach and ammonia or hydrochloric acid (salfuman), because its mix causes a release of chlorine, which is toxic.
- Label properly all the household cleaning.
- Do not pulverize insecticides and garden products on the people, foods or domestic animals.
- Protective mask should always be worn when spray paints, insecticides are used.
- Wash your hands with abundant water after using any chemical product.
- Do not stay in rooms that have currently been painted or varnished.
- Do not stay in rooms treated with insecticides.
- Do not keep the car started inside small garages or places that are not well ventilated.
- Do not use stoves or braziers in the rooms.
- Close the gas valve when is not used and at night.
- In case of noticing gas smell, do not use electrical outlets, lighters or matches.
- Do not eat foods which are not properly refrigerated.
- Do not eat canned foods that are dented, perforated or expired.
- Discharge canned foods that after opening release strange products.

- If poison is an acid or alkalis (bathroom cleaners, chlorine, bleach, detergents and wash products).
- If poison is a product derived from petroleum (gasoline, kerosene, thinner, floor waxes, etc.).

WHAT TO DO IN CASE OF ALCOHOL POISONING

In case of finding an individual who has drunk alcohol and has vomit, loss of consciousness, shakes, etc., it might be an alcohol poisoning.

In this case is necessary to follow the next steps:

- Transfer the individual to the emergency room, where the patient will be rehydrated and will be given vitamin B_6.
- Try to clothe the intoxicated because does not have to suffer cold. This is important because people intoxicated with alcohol poisoning do not have a regulation of the body temperature.
- If going to the emergency room, the intoxicated vomits, keep the victim lying down to avoid he might drown with his own vomit.
- Keep the intoxicated person awake.
- If the intoxication is not severe, the person has a deep discomforts and vomiting, he should be kept hydrated and resting in a cool place and quiet until the alcohol effects have passed, it commonly happens between 12 and 24 hours after drinking alcohol.

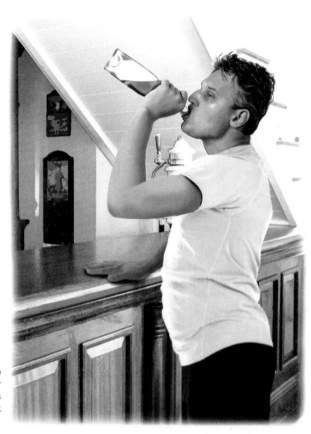

Alcohol might be toxic and trigger serious problems if it is not drunk with caution.

LEVELS OF ALCOHOL POISONING

INTOXICATION LEVEL	ALCOHOL LEVEL IN THE BLOOD	SYMPTOMS
• First level	• 0,5-0,8 mg/100 ml (3 shots of whiskey or 5 beers)	• Lack of coordination • Verbiage • Euphoria • Lack of fatigue sensation • Increased reflex sensation
• Second level	• 8-1,5 g/1.000	• Verbiage • Impulsivity • Disinhibition • Irritability • Inconsistent movements
• Third level	• 1,5-4 g/1.000	• Aggressive attitude • Confusing language • Difficulty to maintain the balance
• Fourth level	• 4 g/1.000	• Depression of the central nervous system • Death

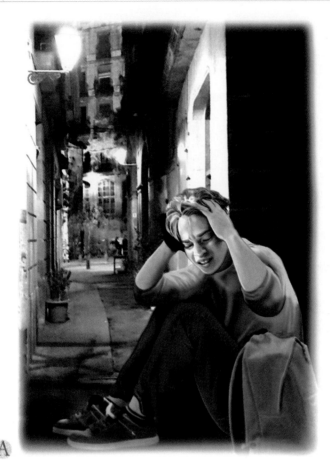

A

An excessive consumption of alcohol, in addition of causing drunkenness, will cause a hangover (nausea, headache, stomachache, general discomfort, etc.). That is why is very important to be responsible before alcohol consumption and, in case of exceeding it, take the appropriate measures to minimize the consequences.

Toxic inhalations

Carbon monoxide poisoning

- Carbon monoxide is a colorless, odorless and tasteless gas that frequently pro-
duces deaths as a consequence of its toxicity. The associated accidents to carbon

---

REMEDIES AGAINST HANGOVER

- The symptoms associated to the hangover such as nausea, headache, heartburn and generalized tiredness, they are commonly relieved in 24 hours approximately. The next advices might be followed in order to treat to reconstruct the body after the exaggerated alcohol consumption:
  - It has been demonstrated that fructose which appears in the fruits, helps to eliminate alcohol from the body relatively quickly. In case of alcohol poisoning, it is recommended fruit juice and honey consumption.
  - Drink much water to restore the dehydration caused by alcohol.
  - Soups and consommés have relieving effects on the digestive system and replenish the mineral salts lost.
  - In case of headache, it is recommended to take orally pain relievers such as paracetamol or aspirin.
  - Rest and sleep for as long as is necessary.

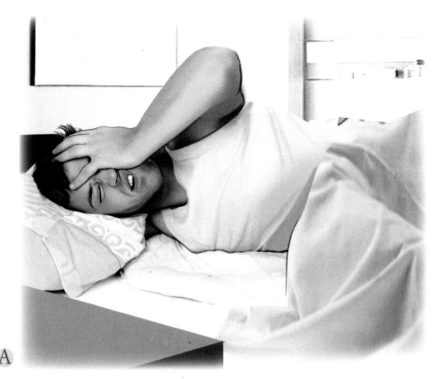

When you are at home, especially sleeping, you must make sure that all the natural gas facilities are closed to avoid emanations that could be fatal.

ASSOCIATED SIMPTOMS TO INTOXICATION BY CARBON MONOXIDE

- Headache.
- Dizziness.
- Nausea.
- General weakness and lose of conscious.
- Inability to concentrate or moving properly.
- Chest pain.
- Difficulty breathing.
- Seizures.
- Coma.

monoxide mainly occur at home, during cold seasons, at nights while victim is resting. This gas is produced through any source of heating or fire without proper ventilation and in the same way is found into the emanating gases by exhaust pipes of motor vehicles.

HOW TO DEAL WITH A SUSPECTED INTOXICATION CAUSED BY CARBON MONOXIDE

- Take the victim to an open place, working to ensure that he/she breaths fresh air.
- Keep the airway open.
- Loosen tight-clothing, mainly around neck and abdomen to improve the breathing pattern.
- Look for medical assistance as a matter of priority, even if the victim recovers successfully. Get in contact with your emergency local number or transfer the victim to the nearest emergency service.

WHAT TO DO WITH INTOXICATION THROUGH THE RESPIRATORY TRACT

- General rules:
  - First of all, the injured should be taken from the place where it has been produced the intoxication and, if it is possible, take the victim to a ventilated place.
  - Before removing the injured from the toxic environment, it should be taken into account that the person who help the victim, should be protected from the toxic environment, whether with a mask or with a wet towel on the mouth or nose.
  - Transfer immediately the patient to the emergency room.
- Inhalation of toxic gases:
  - The most common causes of inhalation of toxic gases are:
    - The leaks of butane gas, at home or in poor ventilated places. Fortunately these gases release a characteristic smell which facilitates its detection.
    - Sometimes the stoves and heaters that do not work correctly and release monoxide carbon, which is a very dangerous gas, because does not release smell, does not irritate the mucosa, for this reason is very difficult to detect it.
    - Released gases by cars in closed places (garages, workshops, small rooms and well not ventilated). This case is very dangerous because the exhaust pipe of the car also releases carbon monoxide. Nevertheless, the exhaust pipe might also release smells that come from other kind of gases, so that they are easily detected.
- Carbon monoxide intoxication:
  - The carbon monoxide is a colorless, odorless and insipid gas.
  - This gas is released by incomplete combustion of stoves that do not properly work, by the smoke of the cigarettes and by the exhaust pipes of the cars.
  - The intoxication by this gas is produced in room without ventilation, in tunnels, closed garages and in kitchens with gas stoves without ventilation.
  - This intoxication is very dangerous because might cause death, if the people sleep in a room without ventilation with gas heater that do not work correctly.
  - When the injured person is conscious, the symptoms that cause this intoxication are: reflexes reduction, severe headache, vomiting, etc.
  - If the injured is unconscious, he will have the next symptoms:
    - Floppy arms and legs and without strength.
    - Difficulty breathing.
    - Skin that becomes pink.
    - Lack of flickering.
  - If it is suspected that the injured is intoxicated by carbon monoxide, he will be immediately taken out from the room where is the victim and transfer to a ventilated place.
  - If the victim does not breathe, it will be necessary to practice cardio respiratory resuscitation.
  - Take the injured to the emergency room.

- At home, all implements that work with gas also are source of carbon monoxide, as well as rotisseries that use charcoal or chemical fuels.

HOW TO PREVENT CARBON MONOXIDE INTOXICATIONS

- Install carbon monoxide detectors in each floor at home, especially in rooms where most of the family sleeps.
- Make sure that all appliances present a proper installation, ventilation and maintenance.
- Performs preventive maintenance every year of all appliances shown at home.
- Do not use fuels (gas, industrial alcohol, kerosene) in close places or confined. Never use a rotisserie within the household.
- Make sure that space heaters have proper ventilation.

ACUTE INTOXICATION CAUSED BY LSD AND HALLUCINOGENS

- Hallucinogenic substances are able to cause disorders of the perception and senses, causing hallucinations. Drug user might think that these hallucinations are real and in some cases may cause panic and terror.
- The hallucinogenic substances might be found in the nature, such as the psilocybin of some mushrooms, the mescaline which contains the peyote mushroom, or those substances might synthesized in laboratories, such as LSD (lysergic acid diethylamide), or the PCP (phencyclidine), that is called angel dust.
- The hallucinogens consumers experience perception alterations, in the form of visual and auditory hallucinations.
- It is not common to have intoxications or overdoses caused by hallucinogens substances. However, given that hallucinations might cause terror and panic to the consumer, what is commonly called as a "bad trip", accidents related with these hallucinations might occur.
- Therefore, the consumer should be treated calmly, avoid the consumer from injuring himself and keep him in a lighted place that does not allow him to have more hallucinations.
- After that, the intoxicated will be moved to the emergency services to receive the appropriate medication and avoid complications.

- To rescue an individual who is suspected of being victim of intoxication by carbon monoxide, the person who is helping with the rescue must be extremely cautious to avoid being also a victim of this gas.
- Before getting into a place with a potential victim, is important to take 2 or 3 deep respirations and in the previous instant take enough air keeping it inside lungs to avoid breathing carbon monoxide in the place which allegedly is found its presence in considerable amounts.
- It must be near the floor (where its concentration is lower) crawling if necessary. When getting into the place, limit yourself to remove the victim.

ASSOCIATED COMPLICATIONS TO TEMPERATURE AND ENVIRONMENTAL CONDITIONS

Exposure to cold

Freezing

- Freezing of some parts of the body can be given as consequence of exposure to very low temperatures. Freeze is produced when forming ice crystals inside skin cells

ASSOCIATED SYMPTOMS TO FREEZING
• Redness, burning pain, burning, stabbing.
• White skin that after change to a grayish tone. Waxy skin, inflammation, edema.
• Cold and drowsiness.
• Absence of pain in advance stages.
• Blisters.

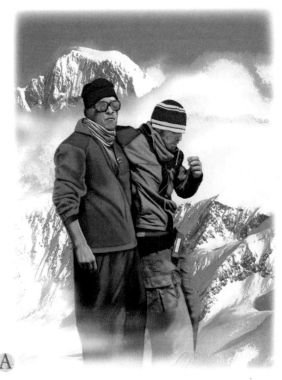

You should not go on a trip to a very cold place without having all the necessary elements to fight against extreme cold.

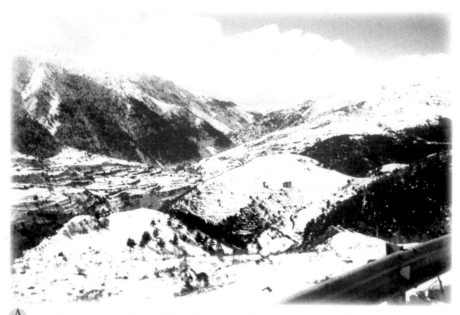

A Excursions and direct contact with nature are highly recommended. That fact must not, however, make us forget that the mountain and weather conditions that might be found there is a danger that many times may have fatal consequences.

and other tissue. The thumbs, fingers in general, nose and ears are the structures more affected. An individual is more susceptible to subsequent freezing to alcohol consumption or if skin is wet.

HOW TO DEAL WITH THE PRESENCE OF FREEZING OF A BODY PART

- Outdoors, cover the affected area with dry clothing, trying to keep it warm. If the affected area is hand, place it in the armpit to increase the temperature. For any reason rub the affected area.
- Enter the victim to an enclosed place, remove wet clothing or excessively cold or any accessory which reduce the circulation on the affected area.
- Restore the temperature of the affected area by the freezing. Introduce the affected area in hot water with a temperature of 38 and 42 °C, it may be used your forearm to test the water temperature, which must be felt hot but it should not burn in the contact with skin. Restore the corporal temperature can last up 30 minutes.
- In the case of not having hot water, wrap the affected area in dry and clean blankets or any other clothing. Do not use lamps or bags with hot water. Do not heat the affected area bringing it to a stove or space heater.
- Apply gauzes or dressings among frozen fingers to separate them of the rest, as far as possible, keep the affected area elevated.
- Give the victim hot beverages. Do not give alcoholic beverages.
- Complete the process to restore the corporal temperature once you observe that skin recovers its color and normal appearance or the affected person shows that is recovering the sensibility. Do not touch or operates the blisters.
- Stimulate the victim to move the affected area as soon as he or she recovers the corporal temperature. In case that the affected area is the low limbs, do not allow that the affected person walks.
- Look for medical assistance as a matter of priority.
- Do not expose the affected area again to the cold until it can be assessed for a professional physician.

HOW TO PREVENT COMPLICATIONS ASSOCIATED TO COLD

- Wear underwear made of polyester instead of cotton; use several layers of lightweight clothing. Wear clothing made of polypropylene, wood or polyester, which adequately isolated the cold.
- Do not wear tight-fitting clothing, particularly socks or tight or fitting shoes.
- Keep hands and feet dry.
- Gloves must not been too tight.
- Do not touch metallic objects with naked skin.
- Do not move or work alone outdoors in weathers extremely cold.
- Avoid dehydration, in cold weathers body requires of an optimum hydration.
- Avoid alcohol and tobacco consumption.
- In elder people, the heater must be established above 22°C/70°F, use electric blankets when sleeping.

Hypothermia

- Hypothermia is defined as cooling of the body to a temperature below 35°C/95°F. Hypothermia usually is the result of an immersion in extremely cold water or for prolonged exposure to an extremely cold weather.

SYMPTOMS OF THE HYPOTHERMIA

- Sudden shakes that cannot be controlled.
- Paleness.
- Muscle stiffness.
- Mood changes in the victim. They might be from hyperactivity and absolute passivity.
- Lack of concentration. The victim does not respond correctly to simple questions and does not pay attention to the given instructions.
- Lack of motor coordination. The victim trips and falls easily.
- Headache.
- Blurry vision.
- The victim might loss of consciousness and go into a coma when the temperature is less than 25°C.
- If the body temperature gets 21°C it is caused a cardio respiratory arrest.

HOW TO DEAL WITH A HYPOTHERMIA CASE

- Get in contact with the emergency local number. Keep the airway open. Restore the circulation or breathing if necessary. *(See cardiopulmonary resuscitation).*
- Place the victim in enclosed place and with a high temperature.
- Remove wet clothing.
- Lay the victim and cover him/her with sheet, blankets or towels to recover the corporal temperature. Do not rub any part of the body which can worsen the harmful effects already presented on the different tissue.
- Give hot beverages if the victim tolerates them. Do not give alcoholic beverages.
- Check specific tissue which may have suffered effects by freezing and treat them adequately.

SYMPTOMS ASSOCIATED TO HYPOTHERMIA

- Trembling.
- Drowsiness, stupor.
- Confusion, sleepiness.
- Muscle weakness.
- Dizzy.
- Nausea.
- Low corporal temperature.
- Loss of consciousness.
- Slow and weak pulse.
- Dilatation of the pupils.

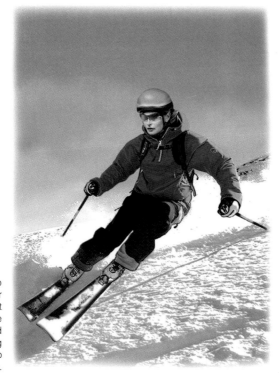

When you go on a trip to the high mountain or it is practiced any sport there, it is indispensable to be properly equipped and have everything that is necessary to face any adversities.

HOW TO PREVENT HEAT STROKE

- Maintain a good level of hydration and drink at least two liters of water every day. It is necessary to drink although the person does not feel a thirst sensation.
- For wearing, wear fine and light clothing, as possible with light colors.
- At home, keep well ventilated the rooms or use air conditioning.
- Do not drink alcohol or beverages that contain caffeine.
- Older infants than 6 months old, they could be taken to the beach, but with high sun protection, at least factor 20.
- The sun block will have to be applied before leaving home.
- Protect the head from the sun, particularly children's head.
- Throughout the day, prepare several light foods, instead one or two abundant foods.

HOW TO DEAL WITH A CASE OF HEAT STROKE

- Remove the clothing of the affected individual and place it in a container with ice or cold water.
- Apply cold compresses and/or alcohol all over the body, especially on the head, armpits and groin.
- Continue the treatment until reduce the corporal temperature under 39 °C.
- Avoid exceeding the temperature decreasing, if temperature increases again, restart the cooling.
- Do not give any medicines, beverages, stimulants.
- Dry the affected individual once the temperature is controlled.
- Transfer the individual to the nearest emergencies service as a matter of priority.

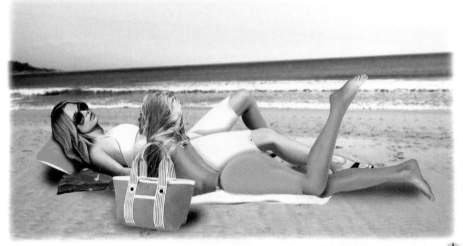

Sunbathe on the beach might be something attractive and rewarding. Somehow you must never forget that sun, although is beneficial, it might also be extremely damaging. It means that sun should not be taken without the appropriate protector and taking the needed cautions. If people do not do like that, sooner or later the consequences will be suffered.

ASSOCIATED SYMPTOMS TO HEAT STROKE

- Corporal temperature over 41°C.
- Strong and rapid pulse.
- Loss of consciousness and confusion.
- Rapid breathing.
- Vomiting and diarrhea.

Heat stroke/sun exposure

- Heat stroke is a condition which demands risk of the affected individual. It is given by prolonged exposure to heat (principally to sun) which alters the corporal temperature for inability of intrinsic regulation of the same.

Decompression syndrome

- Decompression syndrome is shown when a subject ascends of place with high atmospheric pressure at higher altitudes. The principal manifestation of decompression

ASSOCIATED SYMPTOMS TO DECOMPRESSION SYNDROME

- Itchy outbreak, especially in trunk, ears and upper limbs.
- Violet outbreak around waist.
- Drowsiness or pricking around waist.
- Dizzy, whistles in ears.
- Nausea and vomiting.
- Chest pain.
- Difficulty breathing.
- Paralysis.
- Nasal and ears bleeding.
- Joint pain.

HOW TO PREVENT DECOMPRESSION SYNDROME

- Avoid dehydration consuming liquids before diving.
- Make dives in shallow waters.
- Ascend slowly (4-5 meter per minute).
- Avoid immersions at least 4 weeks after an episode of decompression syndrome.

PHOTOTYPES

THE PHOTOTYPES

They are determined by a set of physical characteristics. It may be said that the phototype is the capacity that a skin has to assimilate the solar radiation. According to the type of skin and the result of exposure to ultraviolet radiation or tanning, the phototypes are classified like this: white, brown and black skin. According to the solar burns and the tanning capacity, there are six kinds of phototypes. It is very important that each individual knows which one has in order to take the necessary preventive measures against the solar radiations. These are the most important phototypes:

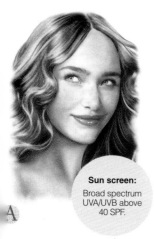

Sun screen:
Broad spectrum UVA/UVB above 40 SPF.

Phototype I

It belongs to a very light skin, this phototype commonly has freckles. It corresponds to the majority of redheads. Their skin frequently burns; it does not tan and suffers allergic reactions to sun. It noticeably flakes off.

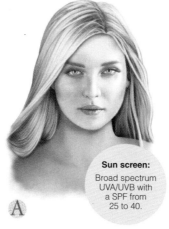

Sun screen:
Broad spectrum UVA/UVB with a SPF from 25 to 40.

Phototype II

It corresponds to light, sensitive and delicate skin. Typically, people with this phototype have eyes and light hair, they almost always burn and they barely tan and significantly flake off.

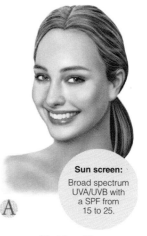

Sun screen:
Broad spectrum UVA/UVB with a SPF from 15 to 25.

Phototype III

People with brown hair and white skin; the skin burns in a moderate way. First it gets red and then gets tanned.

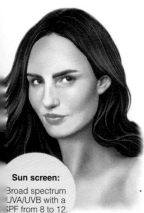

Sun screen:
Broad spectrum UVA/UVB with a SPF from 8 to 12.

Phototype IV

People with brown skin and dark hair; skin barely burns, it is easily tanned right after exposure to sun.

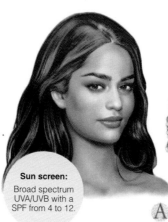

Sun screen:
Broad spectrum UVA/UVB with a SPF from 4 to 12.

Phototype V

Individuals with dark skin that rarely burn and tan immediately.

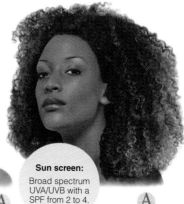

Sun screen:
Broad spectrum UVA/UVB with a SPF from 2 to 4.

Phototype VI

It corresponds to dark skins that do not burn and intensely get tan.

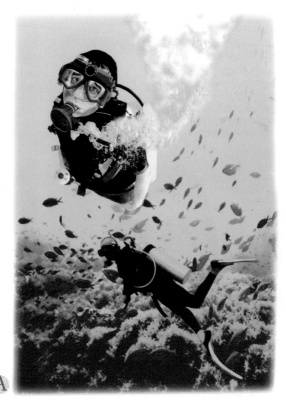

For the sea diving sports, immersion, etc. There is regulation that not only should not be ignored, but also, and over all it should be respected until the smallest detail.

HOW TO DEAL WITH DECOMPRESS SYNDROME SUSPICION

IN A PERSON THAT HAS DIFFICULTY TO BREATHE	IN A PERSON WHO BREATHS BUT IS FOUND UNCONSCIOUS
• Contact the emergency local telephone number or transfer the victim to the nearest emergency service. As far as possible, administer oxygen to the victim. • Keep the airway clear. Restore the circulation and breathing if necessary.	• Place the victim sideways to avoid getting worse the difficulty to breathe. • Contact with emergency local number or transfer the victim to the nearest emergency service. As far as possible, administer oxygen to the victim.

syndrome is the formation of nitrogen bubbles in blood. The presence and travel of an air bubble in the blood can be fatal. This syndrome is principally observed in novice snorkelers and miners underground.

CHOKING, SUFFOCATION, OBSTRUCTION OF THE AIRWAY

Airway obstruction

- The airway obstruction mainly appears when a solid object blocks the upper airway. The main cause of the airway obstruction is commonly food that wrongly does not follow the road of the gastrointestinal system and take the upper airway.
- The Heimlich maneuver is the election method for achieving to unblock the upper airway. The hitting on the upper back, just between the shoulder blades is an alternative option that also may solve this medical emergency, particularly in child population.

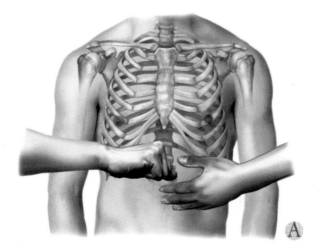

In order to correctly make the Heimlich maneuver is necessary to put the closed fist above the lower breastbone border of the affected patient and with the hand closed press abrupt and suddenly with a soft tendency to lift the patient. The maneuver should be made with strength and repeat it several times.

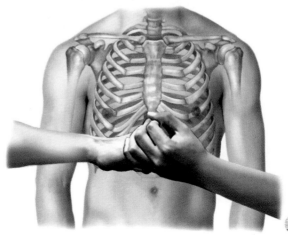

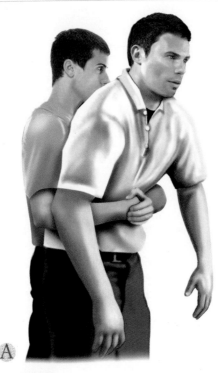

Heimlich
maneuver
in an adult.

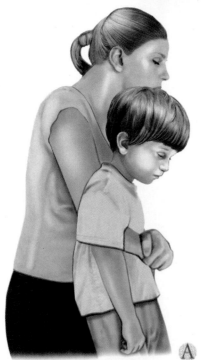

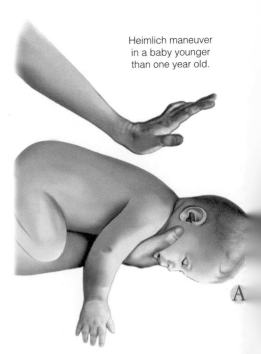

Heimlich maneuver
in a baby younger
than one year old.

Heimlich maneuver in children
older than one year old.

HOW TO DEAL WITH A CHOKING CASE IN A BABY YOUNGER THAN ONE YEAR

General advices:

- Primarily be calm and try that the baby does not get excessively nervous.
- Put the baby on the forearm with the face down and the head lower than the trunk.
- Support the head and shoulders of the baby on the right hand.
- With the left hand, administer four or five strong pats on the baby's back, between the scapulas, with the palm of your hand.
- Verify if the baby has expelled the foreign body by observing the mouth.

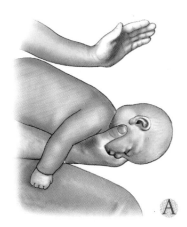

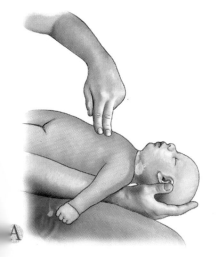

If the baby is able of breathing and coughing intensively:

- Leave the baby coughs, waiting for the coughing reflex to solve the choking.
- Stimulate verbally the baby in order to cough because this is the most effective method for expelling any foreign object from the airways.
- Mean time, call to the emergency service in case of being necessary.
- It should not be tried to remove the foreign body in any way from the airways of the baby, unless the person is sure about it, because might cause the opposite effect, in other words, insert more the foreign body in the airways, causing a complete obstruction of them.
- If after a minute, the baby has not expelled the foreign body and stops coughing, the baby will have to be taken immediately to the emergency room, avoiding moving abruptly.

In case that this maneuver has not been successful, it will be needed to do the next:

Turn the baby and hold him lying on his back.

Try that the baby's head stays at a lower level than the trunk and looking to a side.

Put two fingers on the breastbone and give four or five pats up to the lungs, so that the air goes to the trachea and clear the airways.

Verify if the baby has already expelled the foreign body.

If the maneuver has not been successful, it will be repeated once again.

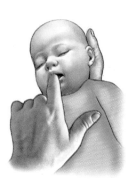

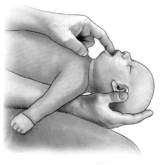

SYMPTOMS THAT MAKE YOU THINK AN AIRWAY OBSTRUCTION

- Heavy breathing or coughing.
- The affected individual normally takes his or her neck.
- Inability to speak.
- Change of the skin coloration (pale or bluish skin).
- Loss of consciousness
- Absent of breathing.

HOW TO DEAL WITH AN UPPER AIRWAY OBSTRUCTION IN A CHILD

- The natural reflex of a child with a strange object in the upper airway is in order to try to expel it through coughing. Do not interfere with this process or insert your fingers in the child's mouth, because this could make that the object is still inserted more.
- Carefully observe the child, try to be calm and keep the child calm.
- If the kid is not able to expel the object, take the child urgently to the closest emergency room service.
- Carry out the Heimlich maneuver if some of the next symptoms are observed:
  - The child takes vehemently the neck.
  - Important breathing difficulty.
  - Changes in the coloration of lips and skin, which could become bluish.

- Put the closed fist (with the thumb toward the chest of the affected individual), just o the lower edge of the breastbone of the affected victim and with the other hand pres sharp and suddenly with a slight tendency to lift the person. Repeat this action severa times until expelling the object that blocks the airway.
- An individual with airway obstruction caused by a normal object involuntarily takes h hands to the neck.

Obstruction of the airways in children

- The children more frequently than adults, swallow strange objects or foods that bloc the airway. A strange object in the airway will cause changes in the tone of voice the child's crying.

ELECTRICAL INJURIES

- The electrocutions are conditions potentially lethal that outside do not show the magnitude of the injury which is presented in the deepest tissues. The type of electricity of the home electrical installation is enough for causing serious injuries. A high voltage power line will be usually fatal.
- The first objective when treating an individual affected by electrocution: do not put yourself at risk. Avoid touching the victim until being sure that is not receiving electrical power.
- All of the electrocutions require urgent medical attention.

SYMPTOMS ASSOCIATED TO AN ELECTRICAL INJURY

- Redness at the injury area.
- Muscle spasms.

HOW TO DEAL WITH AN INDIVIDUAL WHO HAS SUFFERED AN ELECTRICAL INJURY

- Turn off electrical power from the place where the accident occurred or contact the electricity company in order to request for cutting off it.
- For removing the victim from the current, place yourself on an insulating material which does not transmit electrical power (clothing, paper, cardboard, rubber, mat, etc.), and wearing rubber gloves, move the victim from the contact place with a wooden board or wood stick. Do not use any metallic or wet element.
- Contact the local emergency telephone number, keep the airway open and restore breathing and circulation if necessary.
- Cover the injury with a clean and dry garment. Do not manipulate any bag that has been formed on the skin of the victim.
- Verify if there are neck fractures or injuries.
- Take urgently the affected individual to the nearest emergency center in case of having received medical support in the accident place.

EYE, NOSE AND EAR INJURIES

Eye injuries

Chemical burns

- Injuries caused by chemical products on the eyes are a serious medical condition that might become the patient to blindness in case of not being attended urgently. The main chemical burns causes on the eyes are produced by cleaning products, which have to be removed rapidly because the effects may appear if it is not avoided the contact of the chemical agents with the eye (in 1 to 5 minutes).

Traumas in the eyes

- The direct traumas on the eyes with blunt objects require urgent medical support, although the injury does not seem to be serious. The hematomas around the eye might last until 3 weeks to disappear completely.

HOW TO DEAL WITH A CHEMICAL BURN TO THE EYES

- Put the eye or eyes of the affected victim under a steady stream of cold water during at least 10 minutes in order to remove the chemical agent. Make the water runs abundantly from the inner corner of the eye to the outer edge of the eye in order to avoid that the other eye might be affected. The eyelids must remain well separated to allow the water cleans completely the whole eye.
- An alternative option is to insert the face of the victim in a bowl with clean water, with the open eyes and moving them intermittently up and down.
- After washing the eye, close the affected eye and cover it with a clean piece of clothing, gauze or attach it with tape.
- Do not allow that the victim rubs the eyes
- Take the victim to the nearest emergency center.

HOW TO DEAL WITH AN EYE TRAUMA

- Apply cold compresses or ice through a towel on the affected area.
- Keep the victim lying down with the open eyes and the head slightly elevated.
- Take the affected individual to the nearest emergency center.

SYMPTOMS ASSOCIATED TO THE CONJUNCTIVITIS

- Redness of the white portion of the eye.
- White, yellow, green or brown discharge through the eye.
- Sticky Eyelash, especially in the mornings.
- A sensation of a strange object in the eye.

HOW TO WRAP AN EYE

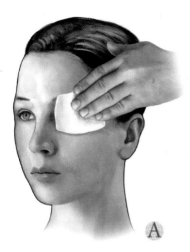

1 After cleaning the eye, protect it with sterile gauze.

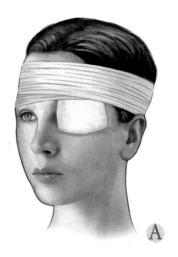

2 With a bandage, give two turns at the forehead level, holding the upper edge of the sterile gauze put in the eye.

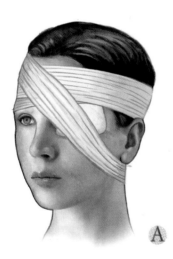

3 Pull the bandage down toward the affected eye, cover it with the bandage and pass it under the ear of the same side.

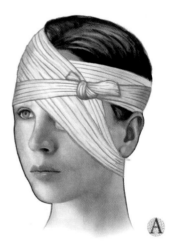

4 Repeat this action until covering completely the whole affected eye.

Conjunctivitis

- Conjunctivitis is a set of eye infections, generally caused by fungus, bacteria or virus. This type of infections might affect one or both of the eyes. Bacterial conjunctivitis is highly contagious and might have prolonged durations, about several days.

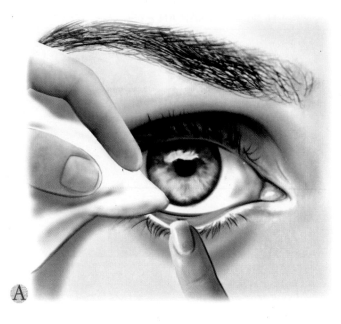

In order to remove and object (hair, sand, etc.) which has entered to the eye, a very clean and fine cloth handkerchief, or sterile gauze.

HOW TO DEAL WITH CONJUNCTIVITIS

- Remove the contact lenses in case that the affected person wears them.
- Consult the physician as soon as possible.
- Apply ice on the closed eyelid by using a towel or handkerchief in order to reduce the pain and/or discomfort.
- Wash carefully the hands after each contact with the affected eye.

Foreign body in the eyes

- The foreign bodies in the eyes might be inserted in the eyeball or they may be seen swimming around the eye. Under no circumstance should you try to remove the foreign body that is found in the eyeball.
- Particles, eyelashes or objects that are observed free in the eye could be removed with many precautions.

Nose injuries

Nasal bleeding

- Nasal bleeding might be as a consequence of a direct trauma on the nose, mucous dryness, infections, dry air or continuous manipulation of the inside of the nostrils. Na-

SYMPTOMS ASSOCIATED TO THE PRESENCE OF A STRANGE OBJECT IN THE EYE

- Pain.
- Burn sensation.
- Watery eyes.

- Redness of the eye.
- Increase the sensitivity to light (photophobia).

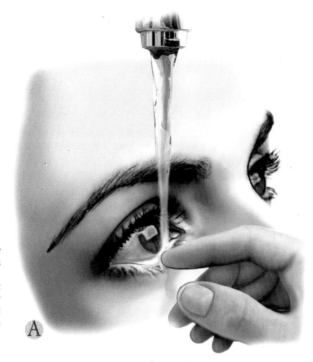

In case that any substance has splashed an eye, it should be put under running water for a while until totally removing the damaging substance.

HOW TO DEAL WITH A FOREIGN BODY IN THE EYE

IF THE FOREIGN BODY IS INSERTED IN THE EYEBALL	IF THE FOREIGN OBJECT IS FREE IN THE EYEBALL
• Wash carefully your hands before revising the presence of the foreign body, do not allow that the affected individual rub the eyes.	• Wash carefully your hands before revising the presence of a strange object and do not allow that the affected individual rub the eyes.
• If it is observed that the foreign body is inserted in the eyeball, do not try to remove it.	• Pull gently the upper eyelid toward the lower eyelid in order to produce tears, which may help to move the foreign body.
• Slightly cover the eyes of the affected individual with a compress, gauze or clothing without pressing it.	• If the foreign body has not been removed, use a dropper with clean warm water or artificial tears and apply several drops on the eye in order to try to remove the foreign body. You might put the eye of the affected person under running water as an alternative. • If the efforts have not been successful, pull down the lower eyelid. In case of observing the foreign body, try to remove it with a wet cotton piece of clothing or with a cotton swab. • Try to do the same previous procedure with the upper eyelid, while the person looks down.
• Take the affected individual to the nearest emergency center in order to look for ophthalmologist support.	• In case of not being able to remove the foreign body, take the individual to the nearest emergency center in order to look for medical support.

HOW TO DEAL WITH A NASAL BLEEDING EPISODE

- Sit the victim with the head bent forward, with the open mouth to allow air circulation to other respiratory tract.
- At the same time press the two nostrils for about 10 minutes at a time.
- Remove slowly the pressure, do not allow that the affected individual manipulates the nose or exhale strongly.
- If bleeding continues, press the nose for about 5 minutes or more.
- Apply ice wrapped in a towel or cold compress across the bridge of the nose.
- Take the affected individual to the nearest emergency room service in case the bleeding does not stop.
- Do not allow that the individual manipulates the nose after stopping the bleeding from 6 to 8 hours.

HOW TO DEAL WITH NASAL BLEEDING IN A CHILD

- Above all, the child should be calmed and given to understand that he could be helped.
- The kid should be seated in an upright position, and lean forward in order to avoid that swallows blood. The head should be leaned forward in order to avoid the possible blood clots inspiration. The seated position reduces the blood supply to head and nose.
- After that, for interrupting the bleeding, a direct pressure should be done on the nostril that is bleeding and against the nasal septum; this pressure might be done during 5 minutes. The pressure should not be interrupted for checking if the bleeding has been stopped.
- Make the child breathes through the mouth.
- Do not expose the child to the sun during these moments.
- After 5 minutes the pressure will be relieved and with this will be proved if the bleeding has stopped.
- After that, ice or cold water compress will be applied in the bridge of the nose.
- If bleeding does not stop, the previous steps will be repeated again.
- If the patient is still bleeding after repeating a couple of times the previous steps, it will be introduced a sterile gauze roll which is wet with hydrogen peroxide, that will act as a plug and it will make the bleeding stops.
- Remove the plug after 4 or 6 hours.
- Do not allow that the child blows his nose.
- If the bleeding is produced, it will be needed to plug and will be needed to the medical assistance service.

sal bleedings in children do not have major complications, while in elderly they migh need support in the emergency service for his control. Recurrent bleedings requir medical assessment to determine the exact cause.

Ears trauma

Ears trauma

- The eardrum may suffer a rupture as a result of a direct trauma, excessive noise infections, related to diving or because of the presence of foreign bodies in the ear.

SYMPTOMS ASSOCIATED TO AN EAR TRAUMA

• Bleeding from the ear.	• Hearing loss.
• Pain.	• Dizziness.

HOW TO DEAL WITH AN EAR TRAUMA

- If the bleeding is the result of a trauma on the head or a skull fracture, it should be a priority this kind of injuries.
- Cover the outside of the ear with a clean piece of clothing or a compress.
- Place the affected individual lying sideways, with the affected side down to allow that blood drain out of the nose
- Look for urgent medical support; take the affected individual to the nearest emergency center.

Ear pain

- Ear pain might be the result of several situations. The infections of the external ear are the main cause of ear pain and among the infections might be named: swimming in contaminated water, is a common cause. The symptoms of the ear infection include the presence of moderate pain, itching and purulent discharge by the ear. Ear infections are conditions that require medical support.

HOW TO DEAL WITH SEVERE OTITIS

- The main objective is to reduce the pain, heal the infection and prevent complication. Generally these types of infections are healed by themselves, without medicine. Some advices might be:
  - Apply painkiller drops on the ear which is sold in pharmacies, without a prescription. Do not apply at cold temperature, it is better warm.
  - Take painkillers (paracetamol, ibuprofen, aspirin) for relieving the pain.
  - In case of being the child younger than two years, or has fever, or the child's state does not improve after 24 hours it will be needed to use antibiotics, but only when strictly necessary. In this case, the physician will be in charge who indicates the most appropriate medicine.

MAIN SYMPTOMS OF MENINGITIS

- Fever and chills.
- Very severe headache.
- Nausea and vomiting.
- Stiff neck.
- Photophobia (hypersensitivity to the light).
- Decrease of the conscious state.
- Rigidity of the neck.
- Fast breathing.
- Sometimes, skin spots.
- Kernig meningitis symptoms
- Brudzinski meningitis symptoms.

HOW TO DEAL WITH A FOREIGN BODY IN THE EAR

- Foreign bodies in the ears, especially those that are very small, have to be removed by an experienced health professional. In case of having in the ear a piece of cotton or paper, it could be removed with tweezers. However, after removing it, consult the physician in order to confirm that the foreign body has been completely removed.
- Do not apply water or oil in the eye to remove the foreign body. The foreign bodies might be diluted, expanded or vanished by the liquids, which will make difficult to remove the object.
- The only situation in which could be justified the use of oil is when there is a live insect in the ear; the mineral or olive oil might kill the insect. Consult the nearest emergency service in order to achieve a definitive extraction.

- Ear pain is also frequently related to throat and respiratory infections, which cause middle ear infections. The symptoms of the otitis media include pain, fever and sometimes discharge by the ear.
- Do not insert cotton swabs or other objects in the ear when the pain appears or when infection is suspected. Consult urgently to the physician.

Foreign body in the ear

- The presence of foreign bodies in the ear is frequent among children because they commonly insert several objects there. Sometimes insects might be another cause of foreign bodies in the ears.

TEETH INJURIES

Injuries in the teeth

- The traumas on the teeth that cause their loss will have about 30 minutes for being implanted again.

HOW TO DEAL WITH A TOOTH LOSS

- Wash the tooth with cold water, do not apply soap. Keep the tooth on the space where it was removed by using gauze or a clean piece of clothing.
- The alternative option is place the tooth on a bowl with milk or saliva until the patient is attended by a dentist that implants it again.
- Control the bleeding by pressing the wound with gauze or a clean piece of clothing.
- Take the individual to the nearest odontology emergency room.

TRAUMAS TO THE HEAD

Head injuries

- Head injuries should be taken as potentially dangerous, because they might be life threatening. The main causes of head injuries are: falls, a sharp blow to the head and car accidents. Individuals with head injuries might also have neck injuries.

SYMPTOMS ASSOCIATED TO A HEAD INJURY

- Cut, scrape, inflammation, bump, or depression on the head's area.
- Confusion, consciousness loss, dizziness.
- Nose, ears or mouth bleeding.
- Crystalline discharge from the nose or ears.
- Paleness or ruddy face.
- Headache.
- Vomitting.
- Difference size in the pupils.
- Anxiety.
- Speaking difficulty.
- Convulsions.

HOW TO DEAL WITH A HEAD KNOCK

- Keep open the airway. Manage the situation with precaution at the possibility of a cervical injury.
- Keep the person lying down and keeping the body temperature.
- Do not give foods or drinks to the affected individual.
- Be aware of behavior changes and the alert status of the affected individual.
- Be careful and give the first aids to the current bleedings.
- Take the individual to the nearest emergency center, putting pieces of clothing, towels or sheet to each side of the head in order to avoid that it moves from one side to another.
- Do not remove the helmet in case that the person who has the accident, wears it. The only reason for removing the helmet is that the individual needs cardiopulmonary resuscitation or when a bleeding wound might be under the helmet and it has to be controlled.

SYMPTOMS ASSOCIATED TO A NECK INJURY

- Headache.
- Neck stifness.
- Inability for moving the limbs.
- Inability for moving some parts of the body.
- Loss of the sensitivity on the limbs or tingling sensation in arms and legs.

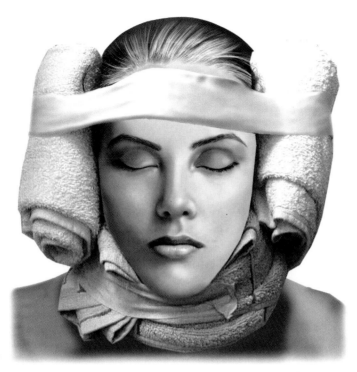

Neck immobilization when a neck injury is suspected.

HOW TO DEAL WHEN A NECK INJURY IS SUSPECTED

WHEN IT IS INDISPENSABLE TO MOVE THE VICTIM BECAUSE OF THE RISK THAT REPRESENTS FOR HIS OR HER LIFE

- Immobilize the individual's neck, tying a towel or a piece of clothing to each side of the neck, avoiding that the immobilization interferes with breathing. As much as possible use a wooden board that cover the back of the individual's body from the neck until the buttock area.
- Keep open the airway; restore breathing and circulation in case of being necessary.
- Contact urgently the emergency center.
- As possible, limit the neck movement of the affected individual.
- Keep the body temperature of the individual with blankets, dry clothing until might be supported by a health professional.

Neck injuries

- Neck injuries must be suspected when there are head injuries. There is absolutely no reason to try to move an individual who is suspected of having a neck injury, at least the fact of not moving the victim might be life threatening.

ABDOMINAL PAIN AND GASTROINTESTINAL DISORDERS

Abdominal pain

- The causes of abdominal pain are multiple: sometimes representing important medical problems which might need immediate medical attention.
- The abdominal pain in children is common; being generally with little medical importance at least is prolonged more than an hour and/or is accompanied by another symptom.
- For both adults and children if the symptoms are severe or persistent, it is important to look for medical support urgently. An individual with severe abdominal pain should not be treated with enemas, medicines, foods, of laxatives liquids (including water) without medical support, because this type of actions might worsen the situation, cause a complication or alter the medical or surgical treatment.

Abdominal pain in adults

- An adult with abdominal pain associated to any of the next conditions, should receive urgent medical support in a hospital:
  - Current abdominal surgery or current endoscopy
  - Severe pain located in a specific abdomen area.
  - Pain that is started diffusely (non localized) and which later on is localized or is moved to the lower right side of the abdomen.
  - Abdominal pain which is produced radiated or is moved toward the back or the shoulder.
  - Abdominal pain with fever, sweating, bleeding in the stools, dark stool (black) or bleeding in the urine.
  - Abdominal pain which is suddenly severe and non tolerable or which makes the person to wake up from the deep sleep.
  - Severe pain in the lower back (lumbar region) or side (in the flank) which is spread or is spread in the groin.
  - Abdominal pain during pregnancy or is related to an abnormal vagina bleeding.
  - Abdominal pain with dry mouth and mucus (dry skin, dry eyes), sunken eyes, dizziness sensation when having a standing position, decrease of the frequency and amount of urine (dehydration symptoms).
  - Abdominal pain related to breathing difficulty.
  - Pain associated to a trauma, hitting or abdominal wound.
  - Abdominal pain with blood vomiting or dark green or brown vomiting.

SYMPTOMS OF DIARRHEA IN ADULTS

- Increase of the number of stools, decrease of the consistency and changes of coloration in the stools (more clear stools).
- Abdominal cramps.
- Tiredness, generalized weakness.
- Thirst.
- Presence of blood pintas in the stool.

Abdominal pain in children

- Small kids with abdominal pain commonly cry intensively, bend the legs taking the knees toward the chest, having a fetal position. A child should be taken to the emergency service in case of having one of the next conditions:
  - Strong vomiting (bullet), after receiving foods in infants of 3 or 6 months of age.
  - Abdominal pain which suddenly appears disappears and later on reappears without any notice.
  - Abdominal pain with red jelly stools, blood in the stools or stools with mucus and/ or foamy.
  - Abdominal pain with green/brown vomiting.
  - Pain related to swollen or distended abdomen that when is touched, is felt harder than normal.
  - Pain associated to the presence of hard masses in the scrotum, groan or lower abdomen.

Diarrhea

- Diarrhea is defined as frequent stools and generally with a watery consistency (less consistent than usual) and it has several causes. The main identified causes are: food intoxication, secondary effects of the medicines, emotional stress and gastrointestinal infections both viral and bacterial.
- The main factor to determine is the orally tolerance. Sometimes diarrhea might be related to vomiting, that is why intolerance to liquids intake orally might trigger rapid dehydration and could be necessary to hospitalize the individual. In case that the oral tolerance is right, the diarrhea might be treated more easily.

Diarrhea in adults

- The presence of dehydration signs should be taken as an alarm signal and the affected individual must be taken to the emergency service.

HOW TO DEAL WITH DIARRHEA IN ADULTS

- Give only a liquid diet to restore the loss liquids as a result of the stools. Prepare a rehydrated solution in case of not having one of them. Give 250 ml of the solution every hour.
- In case that diarrhea lasts more than two days or the amount of urine decrease, consult to the nearest emergency service because of the dangerous dehydration risk.

DEHYDRATION SIGNS ASSOCIATED TO DIARRHEA

- Presence of the 3 or more watery stools in intervals of 4 to 6 hours.
- Fever.
- Dry mucus, dry mouth.
- Decrease in the frequence and amount of produced urine.
- Dizziness, weakness.
- Sunken eyes.
- Vomiting.
- Presence of mucus or blood in the stools.
- Black/dark stools.
- Weak crying in kids.
- Prolonged and frequent abdominal cramps.

Diarrhea in children

- The main causes of diarrhea in kids are the infections, contamination or food intoxication, allergies or intolerance to the foods, laxative effects of food and poisoning.
- The tolerance to the liquids intake is important for determining the severity of the diarrhea. If the child tolerates liquids, it is likely that the diarrhea is mild and might be possible to recover the loss liquids. On the opposite and with the presence of vomiting, it is probable that the kid dehydrates rapidly, for this reason is necessary to take

HOW TO DEAL WITH VOMITING?

- Try to rest and stay in bed.
- Drink liquids in small amounts in order to keep the body hydration level and avoid dehydration.
- If the patient is a baby, as soon as possible, the best is to give breast feed.
- The babies that are fed with a baby bottle should drink the prepared liquid a little bit diluted.
- Much liquid should not be drunk at a time because it could cause a contrary effect when stretching the stomach walls and giving place to a new vomiting.
- If vomiting is continuous, it will be needed to call the physician, because it might be the sign of a more serious pathology.

APPROPRIATE DIET IN CASE OF CONSTIPATION

- If fiber is added to the diet, the intestine is helped to the digestion process and it will contribute to the constipation.
- In order to increase the beneficial effect of the fiber, it should be eaten with much water.
- The main sources of fiber are:
  - Vegetables.
  - Dry foods.
  - Oat bran.
  - Whole grains.
- Other eating habits for avoiding constipation are:
  - Drink more than two liters of water every day
  - Drink plum juice when going to bed.
  - Avoid foods with low fiber such as sugar.

HOW TO DEAL WITH DIARRHEA IN A CHILD

• Give the child liquids to restore them associated to diarrhea and also to restore the electrolytes loss. Avoid giving pure water, fruit juices or milk products. Provide the child carbonated drinks or serums with electrolytes or preparations with carbohydrates and salt solutions.

• Avoid giving solid foods during 24 hours.

SERUM PREPARATION FOR ORAL DEHYDRATION

• 1 liter of water.

• 1 teaspoon of salt.

• 1 teaspoon of sugar.

• 1 teaspoon of sodium bicarbonate.

Dissolve the components by mixing vehemently and give small slips every 15-20 minutes for avoiding the abdominal distension and ensure the tolerance.

the child to the emergency service and in some cases, hospitalization, especially in children younger than 5 years old.

• The main observed symptoms are the presence of frequent watery stools.

CONVULSIONS

- Convulsions are caused by alterations in the electric system of the central nervous system, generating sudden involuntary muscle movements. The convulsions might appear with total or partial loss of consciousness, partial loss of breathing which generally last 1-2 minutes.
- The main causes of convulsions are:
  - Head trauma.
  - Brain tumors.
  - Poisoning.
  - Electrocutions.
  - Stopping medications.
  - Heat stroke.
  - Bites of poison animals.

HOW TO DEAL WITH A NON EPILEPTIC ATTACK OR CONVULSION?

- First of all be calm.
- You should not try to stop the movements of the patient, or hold him, or lift while the convulsion or attack lasts.
- Remove the furniture and objects which are close to the patient, in order to avoid that gets hurt.
- Loosen the clothes in order to breathe better.
- Do not give anything to drink or eat.
- When the incident finishes, place the patient on his side, leaned on the left side and with the head on a pillow. Speak to the victim slowly and with love, in order to reassure progressively the person.
- If the person does not breathe, provide him rescue breathing, while urgent medical support arrives.

ASSOCIATED SYMPTOMS TO A CONVULSION

- Scream or start of crying with short duration and little intensity.
- Muscle stiffness, followed by involuntary and incoherent muscle movements.
- Temporary stopping breathing.
- Bluish coloration of the skin and lips.
- Change of the eyes position, raising drastically the eyes.
- Rapid pulse.
- Loss of the sphincters control (urine and stool).
- Presence of foam or thick salivation.
- Lack of reaction and response to the requests.
- Numbness and confusion when finishing the convulsion.

RECOVERY POSITION OF AN INDIVIDUAL WHO SUFFERED A CONVULSION

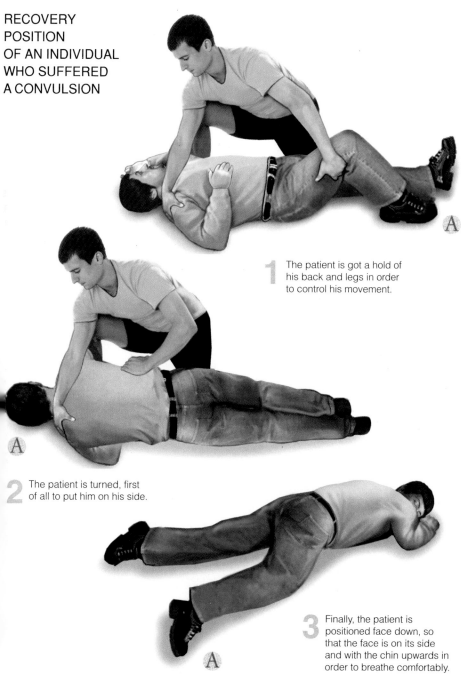

1 The patient is got a hold of his back and legs in order to control his movement.

2 The patient is turned, first of all to put him on his side.

3 Finally, the patient is positioned face down, so that the face is on its side and with the chin upwards in order to breathe comfortably.

Fever.

- Hyperventilation (excessive fast breathing).

- Convulsions frequently appear in individuals with epilepsy, a condition which alters the functioning of the electric system of the central nerve system. Individuals with epilepsy commonly have an aura before the convulsion, which is characterized by the presence of headache, smells, visions or particular sounds which indicate that a

HOW TO DEAL WITH A CONVULSION

- Contact the local emergency telephone number in case the seizure individual has not been identified as epileptic or that a known epileptic has a convulsion that lasts more than 5 minutes.
- Avoid the individual falls abruptly, when observing the fall is starting. Help and place the person in a position in which is avoided to hurt himself or herself.
- If the individual loses breathing and does not recover it rapidly, keep the airway open.
- Make sure the affected individual does not hurt himself or herself, but do not try to hold him for restricting the own convulsion movements.
- Do not insert any object in the victim's mouth; do not put any object between the teeth for avoiding he bites himself.
- Do not throw liquids to the victim to recover consciousness.
- Remove tight clothing on the neck of the affected victim.
- When ending the convulsion, place the affected individual in a recovery position, lying on his side, with the head on one side in order to allow releasing possible discharges that might be accumulated in the mouth and airway.
- Keep the victim lying down for a while after the convulsion for the recovery. The individual may be confused.
- Check the affected individual in order to identify possible injuries such as bleedings or fractures.
- Keep near the affected individual until he or she recovers completely.

HOW TO DEAL WITH A CHILD CONVULSION

- Keep calm; children convulsions commonly produce more panic than being serious.
- If the affected child stops breathing, keep the airway open. Restore breathing in case of being necessary, once the convulsion has finished.
- When the convulsion has finished, place the child in a recovery position.
- Remove the child's clothing and apply compresses with cold water on the whole body in order to reduce the body temperature. Do not apply water directly on the child's face or mouth.
- Contact the emergency center or take the child to the nearest emergency center.

convulsion is about to begin. Most of the individuals with epilepsy easily recogniz these signs.

- Convulsions are considered medical emergencies unless the individual knows th personal history of epilepsy. Convulsions which last more than 5 minutes are cons dered a medical emergency including individuals with known epilepsy, for this, it is priority to transfer the individual to the nearest emergency center.
- The complications associated to convulsions are mainly the hitting that the individu might suffer during convulsion. Do not insert any object in the mouth of the individu during the convulsion because this could affect the air flow and generate choking.

Children convulsions

- Convulsions in children are frequent. The main cause is the fever associated to th presence of severe infections. This type of convulsions are called febrile convulsior and generally last more than 2-3 minutes.
- Convulsions at this age could also be an initial manifestation of epilepsy.

Anaphylactic shock

- The anaphylactic shock is a condition where there is life threatening of the affected individual, which generally causes a severe allergic reaction to the insect's bite, food or medicine.

Traumatic shock/hypovolemic

- This type of shock appears when an individual suffers important blood loss or as a consequence of body liquids loss because of dehydration or diarrhea. In addition might appear for the inability of the oxygen to reach the circulatory system.

SYMPTOMS ASSOCIATED TO THE ANAPHYLACTIC SHOCK	
• Weakness.	• Nausea and vomiting.
• Dry coughing, wheeze in children when breathing.	• Anxiety.
• Breathing difficulty.	• Bluish coloration of the skin.
• Severe itching with the presence of welts.	• Dizziness.
• Abdominal cramps.	• Colapse, loss of consciousness.
	• Weak pulse.

HOW TO DEAL WITH ANAPHYLACTIC SHOCK	
FIRST TIME ANAPHYLACTIC SHOCK	THE INDIVIDUAL HAS ANAPHYLACTIC SHOCK HISTORY AND HAS A FIRST AIDS KIT
• Contact the emergency telephone number, keep the airway open, and restore breathing and circulation, in case of being necessary.	• Help the individual to give the adrenalin's injection. In case of being unconscious, give the injection by following the first aids kit instructions.
• Keep the individual lying down to the side in a recovery position.	• Contact the local emergency number or take the individual to the nearest emergency center.
• Keep the individual calm in a comfortable position.	• Keep the individual lying down in a recovery position unless this position worsens the breathing.
	• Keep the individual in a comfortable position, quiet and in silence.

SYMPTOMS ASSOCIATED TO HYPOVOLEMIC SHOCK

- Paleness or bluish coloration of the skin.
- General weakness.
- Fast and weak pulse.
- Increase of the breathing frequency, irregular breathing.
- Anxiety.

- Increased thirst.
- Vomiting.
- Dilation of the pupils.
- Loss of consciousness.
- Lack of response to a stimulus.

HOW TO DEAL WITH A HYPOVOLEMIC SHOCK

- Contact the local emergency telephone number, keep the airway open. If necessary, restore breathing and circulation
- Identify and treat the shock cause, whether is for bleeding or breathing alteration.
- Keep the individual lying down on the side in a recovery position. Do not move the patient because he or she might have a traumatic brain injury or spinal cord trauma, unless there is a life threatening of the individual, in the position he or she is.
- Elevate the affected individual's legs about 20-30 cm, unless is suspected column or brain injury.
- Keep the body temperature of the patient. Avoid the individual loses body heat by putting a clean and dry blanket above and below him.
- Closely monitor the individual in order to be aware of any change in the consciousness level. Identify the presence of bleeding or fractures and treat in case of having them.
- Do not give liquids or foods to the individual, particularly if is unconscious, has had convulsions, has a head injury, has a deep wound in the abdomen, has been vomiting or has had rectal bleeding.
- As much as possible, look for information about the injury mechanism.

Shock caused by insulin/hypoglycemia

- The shock by insulin appears in diabetic individuals who get confused with the normal dose of insulin and apply more than needed, when the patient does not eat properly or when wrongly take an oral hypoglycemic dose.

HYPERGLYCEMIA AND HYPOGLYCEMIA

SYMPTOMS OF THE HYPOGLYCEMIA

- Sudden onset.
- Lack of attention and confusion.
- Pale complexion.
- Drowsiness.
- Inappropriate responses.
- Headache.
- Sudden hunger.

- Lack of coordination.
- Seasick.
- Tremor.
- Sweating.
- Bad mood.
- Blurry vision.

SYMPTOMS OF THE HYPERGLYCEMIA

- The symptoms may begin gradually.
- Extraordinary thirst and very dry mouth.
- Need to urinate, abnormally different.
- Deep sleep and drowsiness.

- Fatigue and tiredness.
- Breathe that smells like fruit.
- Injuries that lasts to heal.

WHAT TO DO FROM A SHOCK

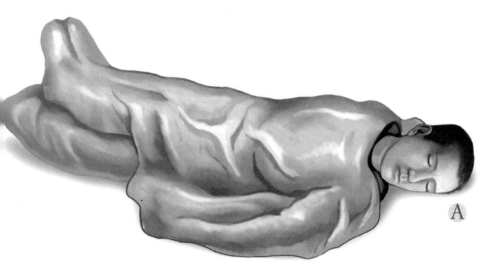

If an injured is in shock (pale, sweats, is cold and has weak and fast pulse), the legs will have to be lifted, will be covered with a blanket and the head will be moved to a side. You have to make sure that the victim does not suffer an injury to the neck.

SYMPTOMS ASSOCIATED TO A SHOCK BY INSULIN

- Excessive hunger.
- Sweating and mucocutaneous paleness.
- Excitation and agitation.
- Shallow breathing.

HOW TO DEAL WITH A HYPOGLYCEMIA CASE?

- If the diabetic has glucose measure equipment, prove the sugar level in the blood.
- If that level is above 70 mg/dl, it will be needed to eat any type of food which has a high content of sugar, such as:
  - Fruit juice.
  - Sugared refreshment.
  - Any candy.

HOW TO DEAL WITH HYPERGLYCEMIA?

- First of all, if the diabetic has symptoms of hyperglycemia, and has a device for measuring the glucose level, he must check it.
- If the level is above 240 md/dl, it will be needed to do a ketone test.
- If there is ketone in the urine, the patient should go to the doctor immediately.
- If there is no ketone it is recommended that continue with the treatment for the diabetes, in order to restore the normal levels of glucose in the blood.
- If the level does not go down, should call to the doctor immediately.

HOW TO DEAL WITH A SHOCK CAUSED BY INSULIN

IF THE INDIVIDUAL IS CONSCIOUS	IF THE INDIVIDUAL IS UNCONSCIOUS
• Give the victim foods rich in carbohydrates (carbonated drinks, water with sugar, fruit juices, honey, etc.). • Take the victim to the nearest emergency center.	• Take the victim to the nearest emergency center.

ASSOCIATED SYMPTOMS TO SEPTIC SHOCK

• Sudden fever. • Vomiting. • Dizzy, confusion.	• Loss of consciousness. • Generalized weakness.

HOW TO DEAL WITH SEPTIC SHOCK SUSPICION

• Contact with the nearest emergency center or transfer him/her to that place.
• Keep the airway open, restore breathing and circulation if necessary.
• Maintain the individual lying down, at rest.
• Avoid the individual loses corporal temperature, cover the person with a clean and dry blanket.

Septic shock

• Septic shock is a condition which might affect the life of the individual, since corporal tissues are not able to use adequately the nutrients and the available oxygen in blood as a consequence of a widespread infection through it, usually bacterial.

SPINAL INJURY

- Back injuries may have final aftermath in the spinal cord, limiting the individual mobility. For this reason do not move an individual who is suspected of having cord injury

HOW TO LIFT AND TRANSFER AN INJURED PERSON

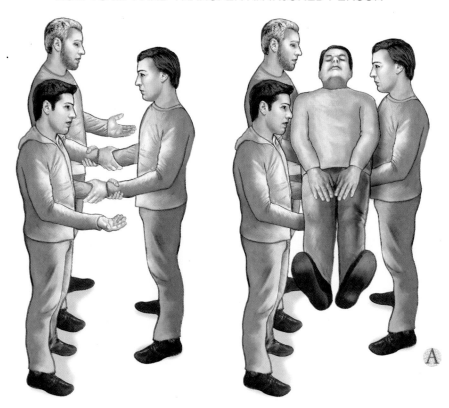

- A person will have to put a hand under the injured person and the other one under the back.
- Another person will have to stand up next to the first one and put a hand under the buttocks and the other one under the knees of the injured person.
- A third person, located on the other side and in front of the other two people, will put a hand under the back and the other one under the thighs.
- In the easiest and most comfortable way, the three people will join their hands in order to make a kind of stretcher.
- So that, moving the three people at the same time, will be able to lift softly the victim and transfer without any problems. The victim will feel comfortable and will not suffer any damage.

CHAIR TRANSPORTATION

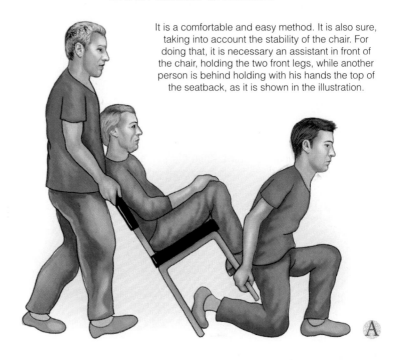

It is a comfortable and easy method. It is also sure, taking into account the stability of the chair. For doing that, it is necessary an assistant in front of the chair, holding the two front legs, while another person is behind holding with his hands the top of the seatback, as it is shown in the illustration.

HOW TO MOVE AN INJURED PERSON WITH THREE ASSISTANTS

- The first assistant will have to put his arms at the height of the gastrocnemius muscles of the victim, the second assistant under the buttocks and the third one under the neck and back.
- The three assistants have to agree about their movements and work together. They kneel and move the victim like a compact and rigid block.
- The three assistants stand up, while keeping the injured with the body toward them.

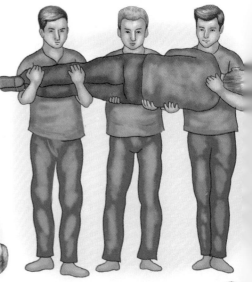

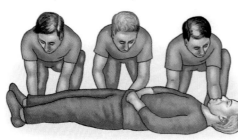

HOW TO MOVE AN INJURED PERSON WITH 5 ASSISTANTS AND STRETCHER

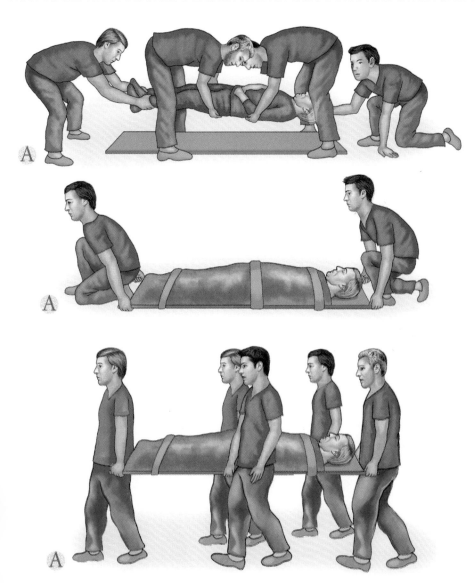

- The stretcher has to be taken to the place where the injured person is located and not the other way around.
- The stretcher will be put on the floor. The victim will be moved as soft as possible, taking into account that always has to be moved like a rigid block.
- Once the injured is lying on the stretcher has to be covered with a blanket because when is immobilized has the risk of reducing easily the body temperature.
- If the stretcher has belts, they will be used because any fall or trip over of the assistants or sudden movements might worsen the injuries of the victim.
- The stretcher with the injured will have to be lifted carefully. Each stretcher handler will kneel in a side of the stretcher and when is in the back of it, and when he gives the notice, all of the assistants will stand up together.
- During the transportation, the stretcher will have to be kept all the time in horizontal position.

THE DRAGGING METHOD

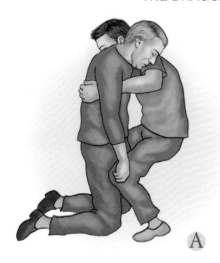

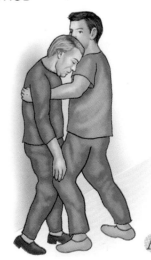

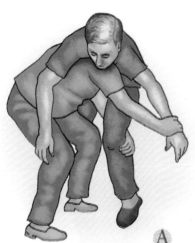

- This type of rescue only has to be used when it is necessary to evacuate and the distance to move the victim is less than 10 meters.
- It only has to be used when the ground is flat similar to the floor. It is not recommended in uneven ground or in stairs.
- The method to follow is the next:
  - The rescuer will be on his knees in front of the victim who will be lying on the floor and on the back.
  - If the victim is conscious, the neck will be surrounded with the hands linked.
  - If the victim is conscious, the hands will be tied with any piece of clothing at the wrists height and they will be put around the neck.

- If it is calculated that the victim's weight is so heavy to drag him, he might be pulled from the feet, being careful that the injured does not hit because of the uneven ground.
- If the victim is light or is a child, he should be loaded on the rescuer's victim:
  - Place the victim on his knees, holding him, and passing your arms under his knees.
  - The victim is lifted and is leaned on the wall.
  - The rescuer has to bend down and drop the victim's weight on his back and putting one of the arms between the thighs.
  - The rescuer has to stand up and hold with strength one leg and one arm of the victim. This position leaves a free arm of the rescuer.

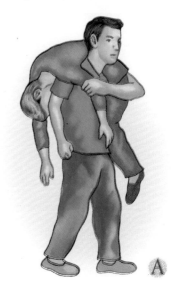

ASSOCIATED SYMPTOMS TO SPINAL CORD INJURY

• Impossibility to move arms, fingers, feet, legs or feet.
• Changes in the sensibility of the affected area, drowsiness, tingling, burn, stinging.

HOW TO DEAL WITH A SUSPECTED SPINAL CORD INJURY

• Contact with the local emergency number.
• Place sheet, blankets or clothing on the sides of the neck and victim's head to limit the movement and avoid it turns up.
• Keep the corporal temperature of individual until medical assistance arrives.
• In case that victim has to be mobilized of the accident place:
  - Immobilize his/her back with a rigid wooden board which covers from the neck until gluteal area.
  - Place the wooden board under the individual keeping the body aligned.
  - Fix the individual to the wooden board by the forehead, under armpits and pelvis by using towels or a set of sheets.
  - Do not allow the victim's body turns, move the patient slowly.
• If the victim does not breath:
  - Tilt the head slightly back to open the airway, but without allowing it turns.
• If the victim is found upside-down:
  - Get the necessary number of persons to turn him/her uniformly until stays face up.

until he/she gets specialized medical assistance, unless individual life is found at risk if he/she is mobilized.

• Spinal injuries may give place to the individual that cannot mobilize the limb, as may be presented with drowsiness and/or tingling of the affected area by the trauma.

STROKES

- The stroke is the result of the partial or complete disruption of the blood flow towards brain. Blood flow disruption can be produced as consequence of the presence of a blood clot in a blood vessel, by the narrowing or blood vessel rupture which takes blood to brain. Strokes should receive urgent medical assistance to reduce the probability of permanent brain damage and aftermath.

ASSOCIATED SYMPTOMS TO A STROKE ACCIDENT

- Sudden headache.
- Paralysis, drowsiness or changes in sensibility of half body of sudden appearance.
- Loss of speech or incoherent speech.
- Loss of consciousness or confusion.
- Falls or loss of balance.
- Alteration of the vision or double vision.
- Differences in size of pupils.
- Loss of coordination.
- Difficulty breathing, speaking, chewing or swallowing.
- Loss of sphincters control (urine and involuntary bowel).

HOW TO DEAL WITH A SUSPECTED STROKE ACCIDENT

- Contact to your emergency local number or transfer the individual to the nearest emergency service; the beginning of the treatment is fundamental to reduce the risk of aftermath.
- Keep the airway open.
- Place the individual on the affected side, on his or her side
- Keep the individual calm.
- Apply cold compresses on the head of the affected individual.

HOW TO DEAL WHEN A TRANSIENT ISCHEMIC STROKE IS SUSPECTED

- Contact with the local emergency number or transfer the individual to the nearest emergency service; The beginning of the treatment is essential to reduce the risk of aftermath.
- Keep the airway open.
- Place the individual on the affected side, on his side.
- Keep calm the individual.
- Apply cold compresses on the head of the affected individual.

ISCHEMIC STROKE ACCIDENT

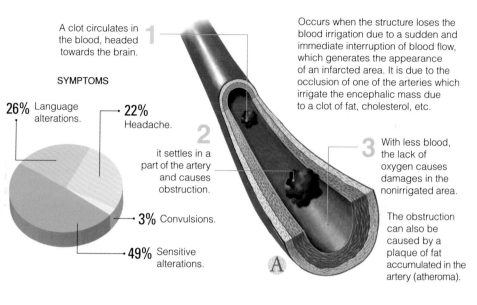

A clot circulates in the blood, headed towards the brain. **1**

Occurs when the structure loses the blood irrigation due to a sudden and immediate interruption of blood flow, which generates the appearance of an infarcted area. It is due to the occlusion of one of the arteries which irrigate the encephalic mass due to a clot of fat, cholesterol, etc.

SYMPTOMS

26% Language alterations.

22% Headache.

2 it settles in a part of the artery and causes obstruction.

3 With less blood, the lack of oxygen causes damages in the nonirrigated area.

3% Convulsions.

49% Sensitive alterations.

The obstruction can also be caused by a plaque of fat accumulated in the artery (atheroma).

HEMORRHAGIC STROKE ACCIDENT

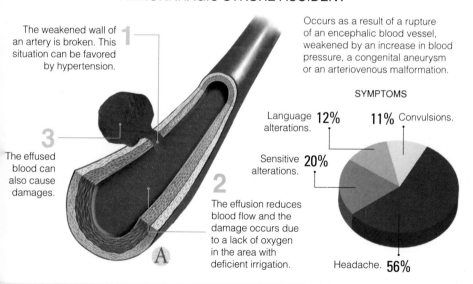

The weakened wall of an artery is broken. This situation can be favored by hypertension. **1**

Occurs as a result of a rupture of an encephalic blood vessel, weakened by an increase in blood pressure, a congenital aneurysm or an arteriovenous malformation.

SYMPTOMS

Language **12%** alterations.

11% Convulsions.

3 The effused blood can also cause damages.

Sensitive **20%** alterations.

2 The effusion reduces blood flow and the damage occurs due to a lack of oxygen in the area with deficient irrigation.

Headache. **56%**

ASSOCIATED SYMPTOMS TO TRANSIENT ISCHEMIC STROKE

- Mild mental confusion.
- Light dizziness.

- Difficulty speaking.
- Muscle weakness.

Transient ischemic stroke

- Transient ischemic strokes are partial occlusions and reversible of blood circulation to brain. Frequently is presented in elderly adults between 50 to 70 years and the symptoms are fully resolved after 24 hours.

HEART ATTACK

- Heart attacks are conditions which rapidly may involve individual's life that is why they must be treated as emergencies. Heart attacks (myocardial infarction) appear when blood flow through arteries (coronary) which brings the blood to heart muscle is not

ASSOCIATED SYMPTOMS TO A HEART ATTACK

- Pain in the middle of the chest or a permanent hard pressure sensation on the center of the chest, which may last several minutes.
- Irradiation or displacement of pain to jaw, shoulder, arm or back.
- Sweating.
- Nausea and vomiting.

- Generalized weakness.
- Anxiety, distress.
- Mucocutaneous paleness, bluish coloration in lips and nails.
- Difficulty breathing.
- Confusion, dizziness.

HOW TO DEAL WHEN A HEART ATTACK IS SUSPECTED

IF THE INDIVIDUAL IS UNCONSCIOUS

- Contact with the local emergency local telephone number, keep the airway open, restore breathing and circulation in case of being necessary.

IF THE INDIVIDUAL IS COUNSCIOUS

- Contact with the local emergency phone, describing the case and emphasizing about the required oxygen. Transfer immediately the individual to the nearest emergency service in case of not being able to contact the emergency service.
- Place the individual in the sitting or semi-standing position. Avoid the patient lies down totally, as it can make him or her difficult to breathe.
- Administer an aspirin to the individual, making sure that the individual is not allergic.
- Release tight clothes, particularly around neck and chest.
- Make sure the right corporal temperature, covering the individual with jackets or blankets.
- Make sure the individual is calm.

IF IT IS SUSPECTED THAT THE PERSON IS SUFFERING A HEART ATTACK

- Contact with the local emergency phone number, describing the case and making emphasis in the requirement of oxygen.
- Take an aspirin in case that the individual is not allergic to it.
- Place him/her in the sitting or semi-standing position. Avoid him/her lying down totally, as it might make him or her difficult to breath.
- Release tight clothes, particularly around neck and chest.
- Make sure the right corporal temperature.
- Do not take foods and beverages.

HEART ATTACK. SYMPTOMATOLOGY

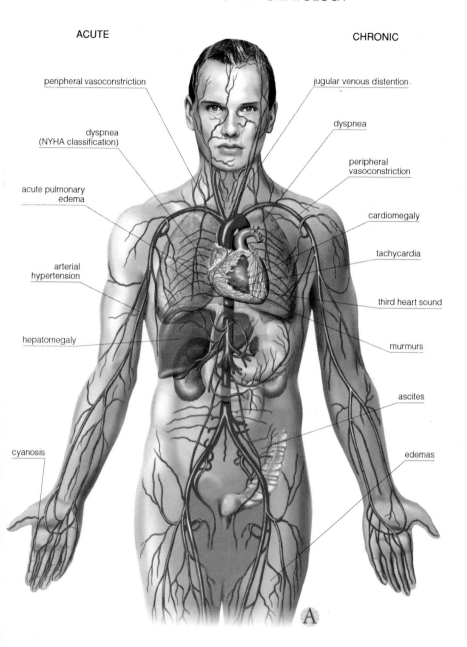

ACUTE

CHRONIC

peripheral vasoconstriction

jugular venous distention

dyspnea
(NYHA classification)

dyspnea

peripheral
vasoconstriction

acute pulmonary
edema

cardiomegaly

tachycardia

arterial
hypertension

third heart sound

hepatomegaly

murmurs

ascites

cyanosis

edemas

A

enough. When the insufficient blood supply is prolonged, a portion of the heart may die (losing its function) or might trigger alterations in the rhythm of the heart beating. The urgent attention of an individual with a heart attack reduces the risk of the heart damage and associated complications.

DEHYDRATION

- Dehydration is the absence of an appropriate level of body liquids (water). Dehydration might appear as a consequence of severe vomiting, heat and excessive sweating, diarrhea and/or food or inappropriate liquids consumption. Dehydration is a

SYMPTOMS ASSOCIATED TO DEHYDRATION	
MILD OR MODERATE DEHYDRATION	SEVERE DEHYDRATION
• Severe thirst which is difficult to overcome. • Tiredness. • Confusion, lack of concentration. • Abdominal cramps. • Difficulty for resting or sleeping.	• Vomiting or diarrhea. • Convulsions. • Weak and fast pulse. • Fast breathing. • Sunken eyes. • Tears absence. • Skin wrinkles in feet and hands. • Dry mouth.

HOW TO DEAL WITH DEHYDRATION
• Put the victim in the shadow, in a zone with less temperature. • Give oral liquids such as water, carbonated drinks, isotonic drinks, gels or liquid jellies. Do not give drinks with caffeine or drinks low sodium. • Look for medical support in case of persisting the symptoms or if there are complications.

DEHYDRATION SYMPTOMS
• Feebleness, fatigue and excessive tiredness. • Thirst. • Dry skin. • Sticky and dry mouth. • Reduction or absence of urine production. • Dark yellow urine. • Sunken eyes. • Headache. • Dizziness. • There is a sign called skin turgor which might help to check the dehydration state of the individual. • When pinching the skin is remains elevated, you have to go to the emergency room immediately because this is a sign of advanced dehydration.

DEHYDRATION SYMPTOMS

- Excessive decay, fatigue and tiredness.
- Thirst.
- Skin dryness.
- Sticky and dry mouth.
- Lack or absence of urine production.
- Dark yellow urine.
- Sunken eyes.

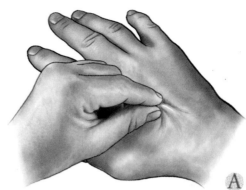

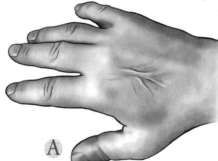

- Headache.
- Dizziness.
- There is a sign named skin turgor that might help to prove the dehydration state of the individual: if the skin is pinched, this remains elevated, it is necessary to go immediately to the emergency room because it is a severe dehydration casea.

medical emergency which requires urgent medical support because is potentially fatal.
- Dehydration is a condition that might be developed rapidly in infants and young children and it is a common condition in elderly people.

LOSS OF CONSCIOUSNESS

- The main causes that should be suspected and assessed from a case of loss of consciousness:
  - Heart attack.
  - Strokes.
  - Bleedings.
  - Diabetic coma.
  - Shock by insulin.
  - Poisoning.
  - Heat strokes.
  - Obstruction of the airway/choking.
  - Inhalation of gases.
  - Severe allergic reactions/anaphylactic shock.
  - Electrocutions.

SYMPTOMS ASSOCIATED TO THE LOSS OF CONSCIOUSNESS

- Absence of response to stimuli.
- Loss of consciousness, location in the time and space.

HOW TO DEAL WITH A LOSS OF CONSCIOUSNESS CASE

- Contact the local emergency telephone number.
- Restore breathing and circulation if necessary.
- If the affected individual normally breathes:
  - Contact the local emergency telephone number or take the individual to the nearest emergency center.
  - Keep the airway open
  - Remove the tight clothing, especially those around the neck.
  - Keep body temperature of the affected individual.
  - Do not give foods or drinks to the unconscious individual.
  - Do not leave alone the affected victim.
  - Keep the individual lying down; do not move him or her unless it is required to make maneuvers for keeping the airway open.
  - It has to be always suspected about neck or spinal cord injuries, for this, the victim should not be moved unless it is strictly necessary.
  - Check the presence of fractures, bleedings or brain injury and provide the first aids.

EMERGENCY DELIVERIES

- A delivery might be in the most unexpected moment, particularly before the expected. In these cases, it could be difficult to take the mother to the hospital. The presence of contractions about two to three minutes apart, urgent pushing sensation (imminent) and observing the head of the baby in the vaginal canal, all of them are signals of an imminent delivery that probably will not allow to take the mother to a maternity ward.

- In case of being possible, allow a doctor or nurse that attend the delivery. It is even useful to contact by phone the doctor in order to receive instructions that improve the conditions for the delivery support. It is essential to keep calm and transmit it to the mother. In most of the cases deliveries occur spontaneously, naturally and without complications.

- For any reason, try to delay the labor, by saying the mother that crosses the legs, refrain the pushing sensation or manipulating the baby's head.

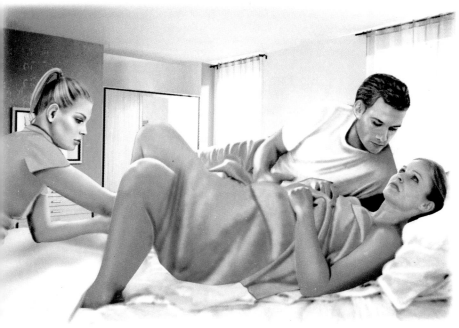

In case of having to attend an emergency birth at home, the laboring woman should comfortably be on the bed with the legs open as much as possible, the feet should be well supported on the bed and below her a big plastic to collect all the effluvia (amniotic fluid, blood, etc.) that will be expelled by the woman.

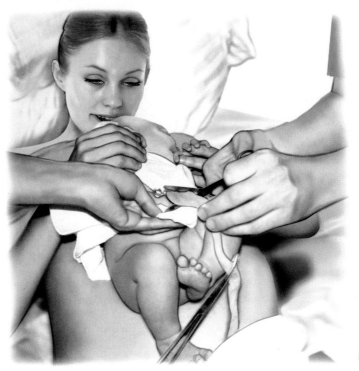

In order to cut the umbilical cord is necessary to use a pair of sterilized scissors, whether by putting them in boiling water for at least five minutes or over a flame for at least 30 seconds. The umbilical cord will be tied with two knots, one of them situated about 3-4cm from its origin in the baby's belly, and the other knot about 5cm of the previous one. The umbilical cord will be cut through the space that is between the two knots.

HOW TO PREPARE THE PLACE FOR IMMINENT CHILDBIRTH

- Put clean sheets on the bed where the childbirth will be attended. As much as possible, put a shower curtain or a plastic sheet under the sheet set.
- If there is no bed, put a sheet set, clothing or newspaper on the floor, under the hips of the mother, extending them until the end of the legs.
- Put the mother face down on the sheets, with the knees bent, the plant of the feet firmly supported on the surface where she is located, with the thighs and knees widely spread.
- Sterilize a pair of scissors or knife by putting them in boiling water for at least 5 minutes or keep them over fire for at least 30 seconds. Once these instruments have been sterilized, put them in a container with boiled water until you use them. This sterilized device will be used at the right moment in order to cut the umbilical cord.
- Near the place of the delivery, there must be the next elements:
  - Cotton clean sheets or towels for receiving and wrapping the baby.
  - Yarns, ropes, strips or clean shoe laces for tying the umbilical cord.
  - A bucket or container for the mother in case she has to vomit.
  - A big plastic bag or big towels for putting the placenta, which will have to be preserved in order to be assessed by the physician later on.
  - Toilet paper, napkins, absorbent paper or tissues for being put on the genital area of the mother after childbirth and the placenta delivery, trying to avoid or control severe bleeding in case of having it.
  - Diapers.

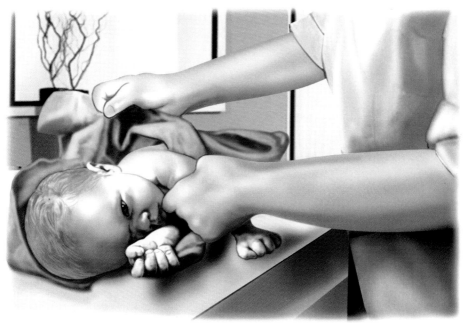

Once the baby is born and the umbilical cord has been cut, the baby will be placed on a table and will be dried with a towel. Place the baby lying on one side because it will ease the baby's breathing.

HOW TO DEAL WITH A DELIVERY

- Carefully clean your hands with soap and water. Do not put your hands or any other element on the mother's groin area. Do not interfere the childbirth or touch the baby's head until he or she has completely left the vaginal canal.
- Once you have observed that the head has surpassed the vaginal canal, guide it for completing the transit outside, covering softly it with a towel or clean cotton garment in order to avoid being exposed to the blood or other secretions.
- If you observe the baby's head is inside a bag full or liquid, try to break carefully that bag with the scissors tip, the knife or your finger, until the whole fluid comes out. Remove the rest of the bag from the baby's face for allowing the baby that appropriately breathes.
- Make sure the umbilical cord is not around the baby's neck. In this case, the umbilical cord might avoid the rest of the baby's body comes out and might limit breathing and circulation of the blood to the baby's head. If the umbilical cord is not around the baby's neck, it will not be a problem and it could be cut later on.
- If it is observed the umbilical cord around the baby's neck, unravel it by introducing a finger between the cord and baby's neck and pass it above the head like if a chain would be removed.
- If the umbilical cord is tight to the baby's neck, it must be cut immediately with care, in order to avoid that the baby suffers as a result of the umbilical cord pressure on the neck.
- When cutting the cord, ask somebody that ties the sides of the umbilical cord with yarn, rope or shoe laces which have already been prepared.
- Keep the support of the baby's head, supporting it on the palm of the hand while the other hand guides it until the baby's body has been completely released.
- Once the head and neck have surpassed the vaginal canal, the baby's body will turn on its side for allowing the shoulders come out. Support and guide this process.
- Hold firmly and carefully the baby. You will notice that is particularly slippery, for this reason, it is important to avoid that the baby slides in your hands. A towel will help to hold the baby in a safe way.

MEDICAL SUPPORT TO THE BABY

- As the baby's breathing is absolutely a priority during the childbirth, hold the baby with the head lower than the feet in order to release the accumulated fluids on the respiratory system thanks to the gravity.
- Softly insert sterile gauze in the baby´s mouth in order to absorb the accumulated fluids and facilitates the baby's breathing.
- If the baby's crying has not started yet, hold him or her by leaning the head lower than the feet, with the face down and gently rub his or her back.
- If the baby does not breathe, use artificial breathing through the mouth and nose of the baby, by keeping the head extended. Make breathings every 3 to 5 seconds.
- Write down the time of the childbirth.
- Once the crying appears in the newborn, wrap the baby in a clean sheet or towel and which is widely long for covering the whole body, including the neck and the back of the head, trying to keep the body temperature of the baby.
- Put the newborn on his or her side, on the abdomen of the mother, with the head toward the feet of the mother and trying that she remains in a lower level of her own feet. It is essential to keep the baby with an appropriate body temperature and breathing correctly. Monitor carefully the baby's breathing and temperature. The baby must not be colder than you.
- It is not essential to cut immediately the umbilical cord. It is ideal to cut it once has stopped pushing (one or two minutes after the childbirth). If it is not possible to take the baby and the mother immediately to an emergency service or to a hospital delivery room, the umbilical cord could be kept intact joined to the baby and the placenta, especially, if there is not a sterile tool for cutting it or until is sterilize it.
- When cutting the umbilical cord which has been previously tied with a yarn, rope or shoe lace at about 10 cm of the baby's body. Tie another yarn at about 5 cm of the first tie and cut the cord in the middle of the two ties. This should be done before expelling the placenta, which will occur in about 5 to 20 minutes after the childbirth.
- Keep the baby warm and near the mother. The body warm will allow keeping the appropriate body temperature of the baby.
- The baby's body has to be leaned with the head at a lower level than the feet in order to release the accumulated fluids in the baby's mouth and respiratory system.

HOW TO ATTEND AND REMOVE THE PLACENTA

- Be patient; do not throw the umbilical cord in order to make the process faster.
- The mother's uterus is kept in contractions which will naturally expel the placenta. This is generally preceded by the expelling of black blood clots. Do not be alarmed for this situation.
- Collect the placenta in a buckle or container for taking it to the hospital along with the mother and the baby. The placenta has to be examined by medical personnel.

ATTENTION OF THE MOTHER AFTER CHILDBIRTH

- Put a cotton piece of clothing, handkerchiefs or a towel in the mother's genital area in order to help blood absorption and other fluids associated to the childbirth.
- In order to control mother's bleeding, put your hand on the abdomen and slowly massage to stimulate the uterus until is felt firm. Continue the two minutes massages every five minutes during an hour or until the mother is transferred to the nearest hospital. If the bleeding is severe, look for medical support urgently, contact your local emergency center.
- Comfort the mother's face with cold water compresses if it is right for her.
- Give the mother small slips of water, rehydration is essential in this moment.
- Keep comfortable the mother with an appropriate body temperature. Cheer her up and make her proud of the good job she just has done.

FEVER AND CHILLS

Fever

- The fever is frequently an indicator of an infection presence and this is a self-defense mechanism for fighting the infection. The allergic conditions such as asthma also may appear with fever.
- The fever episodes with more than 40,6°C always have to give an alarm signal and it is important to look for urgent medical attention in the nearest emergency center.
- The presence of any level of fever in a child is an emergency and medical support to the nearest emergency center should be a priority.
- The average body temperature in an adult is 37°C (+/- 1°C), mild changes are normal, it might be noticed that the body temperature in the mornings the body temperature is commonly lower, and at the end of the day it mildly increases. The body temperature over 39°C is an important alarm signal which must require urgent medical support.
- In adults, the temperature control might be achieved by giving aspirin, acetamino-phen, ibuprofen or any other non-steroidal anti-inflammatory. Remove clothing excess and allow the individual stays in a cool place.

HOW TO DEAL WITH THE PRESENCE OF FEVER IN A CHILD

- There is no reason for giving aspirin to a child.
- Contact a physician before giving any type of medicine to the kid.
- Give plenty of liquids to the child.
- Keep the child resting.
- Apply compresses with warm water on the whole body in order to reduce the body temperature. Check the temperature every 25-30 minutes until is lower than 39°C.

FEVER SYMPTOMS

Fever is commonly accompanied by a series of disorders which are well known as febrile syndrome. Those symptoms are the next:

- Cold sensation (chills) in the initial stage and then heat.
- Redness face and shining gaze.
- Dirty tongue.
- Loss of appetite.
- Tachycardia (rapid heart rate).
- Low urine production, very concentrated and colored.
- Headache.

IN CASE OF FEVER, WHEN SHOULD BE CALLED THE DOCTOR?

Call urgently the doctor if the fever does not come down and it is accompanied of the next symptoms:
- Severe headache.
- Stomachache.
- Ears ache.
- Pain when urinating.
- Severe pain in the joints.
- Difficulty breathing.
- Throat inflammation.
- Vomiting.
- Diarrhea.
- Dehydration.
- Confusion state of the patient (the patient does not know how to answer to questions such as: what is your name? where do you live? What month we are?
- Presence of convulsions.

IN CASE OF INFANT FEVER. WHEN SHOULD BE CALLED A DOCTOR?

A doctor should be called in the next situations:
- If the child has stiff neck, confusion, irritability or drowsiness.
- If the infant is younger than six months or if has any situation accompanied by fever.
- In a 6-12 months old child, if has a febrile process which lasts more than 24 hours.
- Permanent fever above 39,4°C after an hour of starting the treatment.
- Fever that last more than two days.
- Any individual with a temperature above 39,4°C should be examined by the physician in order to search diseases or causative alterations.

HOW TO DEAL WITH THE PRESENCE OF CHILLS

- Keep the affected individual warm, without using sheets or excessive blankets. Do not use bottles or bags with hot water.
- Give hot liquids to the affected individual if he or she does not have nausea or vomiting.
- Look for medical support; it is possible that is developing an infection.

- In children, the temperature ideally should be taken rectally. The rectal reading commonly is more reliable and about 1°C higher than the oral temperature.

Chills
- Chills are nonspecific symptoms that might be the result of many medical conditions such as a common cold, urinary and respiratory infections, food intoxications, allergic reactions and insect bites.
- Chills are a self-defense mechanism which main objective is to raise body temperature. Chills are the result of the reduction of the blood flow to the skin because of the involuntary contraction of the blood vessels that carry it, increasing the circulation to the muscles, which in turn have involuntary and repetitive contractions that try to give heat. Chills are generally followed by fever, which suggests the presence of an infection.

HEADACHE

- The main cause of the headaches is the tension headache which results from the muscle tension in the neck as a consequence of the stress or emotional situations. Other causes of the headache might include:
  - Viral infections.
  - Sinus infections.
  - Allergies.
  - High blood pressure.
  - Strokes.
  - Brain tumors.
  - Head trauma.
- Mild headaches might be treated with acetaminophen or non-steroidal anti-inflammatory such as aspirin, naproxen and ibuprofen combined with resting time.
- Any severe headache that wakes the individual up from the deep sleep, a persistent headache or which is related to other symptoms is a reason for consulting urgently the physician in order to have additional studies.

HOW TO DEAL WITH A MIGRAIN ATTACK

- It is very important to treat the symptoms as soon as possible, because from this depends the pain progression. Generally the individuals who suffer migraine are able to notice the triggering symptoms, knowing the developing pattern of this pathology can thus to be avoided severe pain.
- When the migraine pain has already appeared, the next measures could be taken:
  - Resting in a place free of light and reserved for the noises.
  - In case of having nausea and vomiting, drink much liquid.
  - Place a cold cloth on the head.
  - If the pain is more severe or there are more than three crises in a month, it is necessary to go to the physician, in order to get some medicines which work on the blood vessels of the brain and mitigate pain.

APPENDICES

APPENDIX 1. COUGHING

MAIN CAUSES OF COUGHING

- Cold and flu.
- Nose, ear and throat diseases.
- Pulmonary infections: pneumonia, severe bronchitis etc.
- Chronic pulmonary diseases: asthma, chronic bronchitis, etc.
- External auditory canal diseases.
- Heart diseases.
- Gastroesophageal reflux
- Accidental causes: entrance of foreign bodies in the trachea, smoke, choking, etc.

HOW TO DEAL WITH A COUGHING ATTACK?

- Coughing attack causes anguish in the people who suffer them. First of all, it has to be tried to relax the individual who suffers the attack and advice him that breathes deeply and swallow saliva.
- If the throat itches, candies or pill for the cough might be taken, but they must not be given to children younger than 3 years old, because of the risk of choking. These candies should have honey or an herb that smooths the throat. Candies with menthol must be avoided because it is irritating.
- If the coughing cause is a cold, the mucus will slide from the nose until the throat, and will cause coughing. This situation worsens at night, when the person is lying on the bed. For this reason, it is advised to sleep with the head more elevated than the rest of the body, adding more pillows.
- It is recommended to drink much liquid for diluting mucus and ease the expelling.
- For relieving the sore throat, it will be needed to prepare a hot drink with honey, or a glass of water that is not cold.

APPENDIX 2. ALLERGIES

GENERAL RECOMMENDATIONS TO ALLERGIC PEOPLE

- Allergic people should always have with them the telephone number of their physician.
- Museums generally have higher dust mites than normal, for this reason is recommended to allergic people to go there as little as possible.
- Bus terminals and certain zones of the cities such as squares and wide avenues commonly have high contamination levels, for this reason, those places should be avoided or stay there the shortest possible time.
- It is recommended that allergic people do not spend their vacations in places where they have direct contact with animals such as dogs, cats, chickens, horses, etc. In case of being inevitable, they should not have access to the house where the allergic person stay and even more in his or her room.
- People allergic to certain foods should avoid them, for example coffee, spicy or hot food such as seafood, ketchup, eggs and their derivatives, spicy canned foods and alcohol.
- Very cold living rooms or with air conditioning should be avoided or stay there the shortest possible time because they could irritate the airways.
- Before traveling, the person should go to the doctor and consult about the needed medicine while the trip. The physician will advice the patient if has to continue with the same dose or if it is needed to change it.
- If traveling abroad, it is recommended to get a health insurance with international coverage.

HOW TO DEAL AT HOME WITH AN ALLERGIC TO POLLEN

- Use air conditioning with antipollen filter.
- Keep closed the windows during day hours, when there is greater pollination, in other words, at the first hour in the morning and at sunset time.
- Change your clothes and take a shower when arriving home.
- Remove rugs and carpets from the room of the allergic.
- Remove the big curtains and other objects that might store dust.
- Use the latex or foam rubber mattress or cover it with a special cover for allergic people.
- Keep the house clean.

HOW TO DEAL WITH AN ALLERGIC WHEN IS LIVING WITH A PET

- Keep the animal out of the house.
- If it is not possible to keep out of the house the animal, keep it out of the allergic room and the living room.
- Remove the big carpets and other objects that build up animal hair.
- Remove the big curtains and other objects that might store animal hair.
- Use a latex or foam rubber mattress, or cover it with a special cover for allergic.
- Clean from time to time the animal hair and the places where it is commonly moving.

WHAT SHOULD DO AN ALLERGIC PERSON TO THE FOODS

- Avoid the food.
- Ask for the ingredients of the foods that are eaten. Sometimes any allergen might be hidden in the cooked food. Allergic people to any food should ask about the ingredients when eating in restaurants or out of the house.
- Read the labels of the foods.
- Be prepared for emergencies. The anaphylactic reactions to food might mean life and death, for this reason the people with severe allergies should take medicine for treating the reactions caused by the accidental ingestion.
- Take a bracelet which has written the suffered allergy.

APPENDIX 3. HOW TO USE CORRECTLY AN INHALER

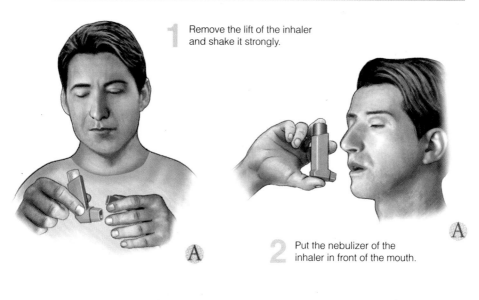

1 Remove the lift of the inhaler and shake it strongly.

A

2 Put the nebulizer of the inhaler in front of the mouth.

A

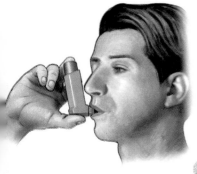

3 Stand up and exhale all the air of the lungs.

A

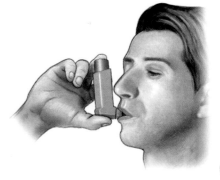

4 Breathe deeply a couple of times and, when you are about to make the third breathing, press the inhaler and start breathing slowly.

A

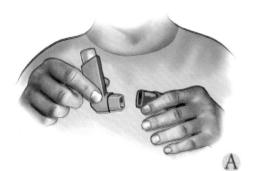

5

In case of being necessary, take a second application of the nebulizer, remove it, wait for about five minutes and repeat it.

A

137

APPENDIX 4. FIRST AID KITS AND TRAVEL EQUIPMENT

HOME FIRST AID KIT

A first aid kit contains the necessary elements to provide an emergency care. It always must be considered that the further the distance to a medical care centre, the most complete will have to be the first aids kit.

• Some advice about the first aid kit location:
  - It must be located in a visible place, and should not be locked because the kit must be accessible inside.
  - The contained of the first aid kit must be made of plastic or metal.
  - All the people who share the same house must perfectly know the place where the first aid kit is located.
  - It has to be revised periodically the expiration date of the material support which are kept in the first aid kit.

• What must contain a home first aid kit:
  - Hydrogen peroxide.
  - Alcohol 96°.
  - Soap or soft antiseptic solution.
  - Cotton.
  - Sterile gauzes.
  - Moistened cleansing towelettes for the hands.
  - Pain killers (aspirin and paracetamol).
  - Antidiarrheal.
  - Laxatives.
  - Antiseptic cream.
  - Cream to treat burns.
  - Antihistamines.
  - Tweezers.
  - Adhesive plaster.
  - Adhesive dressings (strips).
  - Sterile gauze (sized 10 x 10cm), wrapped separately for cleaning and cover wounds.
  - Scissors rounded end.
  - Thermometer.
  - Latex gloves.

WHAT SHOULD CONTAIN A FIRST AID KIT

• Hydrogen peroxide.
• Alcohol 96°.
• Soap or a soft antiseptic solution.
• Cotton.
• Sterile gauze.
• Wet wipes for cleaning hands.
• Painkillers.
• Antidiarrheal.
• Laxatives.
• Antiseptic cream.
• Cream to treat burns.
• Antihistamines.
• Medication for travel sickness.
• Tweezers for removing splinters.
• Roll of sticking plaster.
• Adhesive drapes (strips).
• Wrapped sterile gauze (10 x 10cm) for cleaning wounds and cover them later on.
• Rounded end scissors.
• Thermometer.
• Latex gloves.

ACCORDING TO THE PLACE OF DESTINATION THE KIT MIGHT ALSO INCLUDE

• Tablets for disinfecting water.
• Sun burn lotion.
• Cream for insect bites.
• Cream for local inflammations.
• Activated charcoal for absorbing ingested poisons.
• Sodium bicarbonate.
• Small bottle with ammonia.
• Prophylactics against malaria.
• Antibiotics.
• Oral rehydration salts.
• International Certificate of Vaccination.
• Matchbox or lighter.
• Flashlight.
• Condoms.

WHAT SHOULD CONTAIN A FIRST AID KIT IN A CAR

- If not having water, the first aid kit of the car needs to have physiological saline or hydrogen peroxide for washing possible wounds.
- Alcohol at 96°.
- Soap or a soft antiseptic solution.
- Cotton.
- Sterile gauze or wipes for cleaning hands.
- Painkillers (aspirin, paracetamol, ibuprofen).
- Seasickness pills.
- Tweezers.
- Sticking plaster.
- Box with several dressing (strips).
- Sterile gauze (10 x 10cm), wrapped separately for cleaning wounds and cover them later on.
- Round ended scissors.
- Thermometer.
- Latex gloves.
- Flashlight.
- Clothing triangles for immobilizing and some bandages.
- Thermal insulated blanket.
- Emergency telephone numbers.
- Disposable plastic glasses.
- First aids kit manual.

NEEDED EQUIPMENT FOR THE MOUNTAIN

If you go hiking to the mountain, minimum equipment which protects from the sun, wind and cold should be taken with you, and also a first aid kit. The minimum equipment should be the next:

- Backpack. Should be bit, anatomical and with at least a capacity or 55 liters. The backpack should be tested is the store before using it in order to prevent inconvenience.
- Sleeping bag. It must be of a good quality and must be in the range of at least -5°C.
- Insulated. Choose an insulated bag which protects from the cold of the ground and if it is possible, it should be light.
- Water canteen. It is recommended to take 1,5 liters for personal consumption and avoid dehydration.
- Cane. It is recommended the use of canes that will help to maintain the right balance during the march and will be more comfortable because the cane saves efforts.
- Footwear. It is important to choose good footwear which does not squeeze the foot, or it is very loose. Footwear should be breathable and insulate from water and cold.
- Gloves. You could take polar fleece lining. It is recommended to wear a pair of gloves in case of getting wet.
- Cap. It must cover the ears and forehead. Polar fleece lining is recommended.
- Glasses. The must be gotten in a specialized store. They must have a sun protection better than the normal glasses and a very high UV protection.
- Sunscreen with a high sun protection factor. Snow and sun might cause very severe burns, even more than in the beaches.
- Lip balm.
- Flashlight.
- Pants. They must be comfortable, breathable and which repel water. Cotton or jeans pants are not recommended because they get wet easily.
- T-shirts. They must be comfortable, breathable and repel water.
- Jacket. Jackets with polar fleece lining are recommended because of the dryness capacity and because they are very comfortable for the mountain.
- Waterproof anorak.
- Ski mask.
- Handkerchief for the neck.
- Socks. They should be bought in a specialized store in order to avoid blisters when going to the mountain with regular socks.
- First aids kit.
- Mobile telephone.
- Insulating blanket.
- Candies and dry fruits.
- Mirror for making signs.
- Whistle.
- Water proof matches.
- Map of the area being traversed.

APPENDIX 5. CONDOMS

CONDOMS

- The male condom is a very fine cover that is placed in the penis when is erected. At the time of ejaculation the semen is collected in the condom, avoiding that penetrates into the vagina so that the sperm that contains it could fertilize the woman's egg.
- The condom is a very common method used by the population to avoid sexually transmitted diseases and also to prevent unwanted pregnancies. However, sometimes because of certain movements or imprudent maneuvers during intercourse, or defect of the condom, it could be broken, moved or come off, which will make necessary to use emergency contraception methods, in this case it will be needed to go to the doctor.

SOME TIPS ABOUT THE CONDOM

- It is recommended to have always condoms and enough amounts of them.
- Make sure that these condoms are recognized by the corresponding health authority.
- Never use expired condoms. It is necessary to verify before using the condoms, the expiration date which will appear on the container.
- Keep the condoms in a fresh and dry place, for example in the nightstand drawer.
- It is not recommended to keep condoms in the wallet or in places where the temperature is high because the heat might cause latex deterioration which is the material of the condom.

When and how to use the condom:
- Remove carefully the condom from the packaging, without tearing it with nails or rings, and do not stretch it.
- In order to avoid sexually transmitted infections, the condom must be put before starting the relationship.
- In order to put the condom, the next steps must be followed:
  - Wait until the penis is completely erected.
  - Leave a space between the glans of the penis and the condom so that when ejaculating, the semen is stored in the receptacle that has been created with this space.
  - The condom will be placed on the glans without releasing the tip of the penis.
  - The foreskin is retracted and the condom is slipped through the rest of the penis until reaching the base.
- The condom should be used during the whole sexual intercourse.
- As the ejaculation has been produced, the condom must be slowly removed.
- Do not have to wait until the erection has disappeared to remove the condom.
- When removing the condom, it has to be held from the base to avoid spilling the semen.
- After removing the condom it will be tied and thrown to the trash can. The condom never must be thrown to the toilet.
- The condoms are used only once, that is why they must never be reused.

Why the condoms are broken?
- According to the statistics, due to manufacturing defects only 2 % of the condoms are broken. It means that manufacturing defect is not the most common cause.
- In most of the cases, a torn condom is caused by the use of expired condoms, if the intercourse is violent or the use of a smaller size of the condom.
- The use of non appropriate lubricants might affect the quality of the condom. The use of lubricants based on greasy substances should be avoided. Oils and other greasy substances weaken the latex and reduce in about 90 % its resistance.
- Only the water soluble lubricants are compatible with condoms.

The morning after pill

- In case of a torn condom, it is recommended the administration of the well known morning after pill, as an emergency remedy.
- When taking this pill, composed by a hormones cocktail, it is caused an alteration in the menstrual cycle, avoiding a pregnancy because inhibits or delays ovulation and avoids the implantation of the fertilized egg in the endometrium.
- The effectiveness of this pill is about 100 % if it is taken 24 hours after the torn condom or other risky situation during intercourse.
- This drug must be taken within 72 hours after intercourse and commonly might be administered with medical prescription.
- The treatment is divided in two parts: the first one must be taken within the 72 hours after intercourse and the second dose 12 hours after the first one.
- It has to be insisted the fact that this method only should be used in an emergency case. In any way is recommended as a contraceptive alternative. For that, there are more effective methods and with less secondary effects, information about them could be found at any family planning center.
- Approximately half of the women who have taken the morning after pill experience nausea and one in five vomit. If vomiting is caused after two hours of taking the pill, the dose must be repeated because it has not been still absorbed into the blood stream.
- It must not be forgotten that the post intercourse pill avoid an unwanted pregnancy but it does not protect from sexually transmitted diseases or against AIDS.

Cases in which morning after pill is indicated:

- In case of a torn or slipped condom inside the vagina.
- If the couple uses natural family planning methods and practice intercourse during the pregnancy risky days.
- Problems with the IUD or intrauterine device.
- Ejaculation without condom in the vulva (external female genitalia) or in the vagina.
- When stopping the daily take of oral contraceptives for more than three consecutive days.
- In case of a woman who has been raped.

Cases in which the after morning pill should not be prescribed:

- If pregnancy is suspected.
- If there has been sexually intercourse without any protection before the risky intercourse.

Cases to assess by the physician:

- Women that commonly suffer migraine.
- Women that suffer diseases of the circulatory system and alterations in the blood clot.
- Women that are breast feeding their children.
- Women that suffer any disease of the genital system.

Latex allergy:

- Latex is a fluid with milky aspect which is obtained from the trunk of the tropical rubber tree Hevea brasiliensis. After a long a complex industrial process, it is used for manufacturing rubber. It is also used for manufacturing condoms and gloves.
- Some people, men or women might have allergic reactions when having sexual intercourse. It could be caused due to the use of spermicides along with the condom or with the latex that the condom has been manufactured.
- In order to discard that the spermicide causes the allergy, it is recommended to keep sexual intercourse with several trademarks spermicides. If the allergy reactions disappear, it could be thought that the allergy reaction is caused by the spermicide of a particular trademark.
- If the allergy reaction continues or is more severe, the physician should be consulted and would give alternative protective methods.
- In the market there are polyurethane condoms that reduce the risk of allergy reaction.

WHAT TO DO IF THE CONDOM IS TORN OR REMAINS INSIDE THE VAGINA

- The condoms available in the market are manufactured under strict safety and quality controls, according to health and consumer laws of each country, in view of this can be said that the torn condom is considerably reduced.
- Currently is calculated that the torn probability of a condom is barely 2 %.
- In case of a torn condom, you should go immediately to a family planning center in order to look for advice.
- The visit to the family planning center should be done 72 hours before the incident to avoid the unwanted pregnancy risk.
- In case of not knowing the family planning center or not being available, it will be necessary to go to the gynecologist or the physician.

APPENDIX 6. FIRST AID KIT OF A COMPANY

WHAT SHOULD CONTAIN THE FIRST AID KIT OF A COMPANY

- Hydrogen peroxide.
- Alcohol 96°.
- Iodine.
- Soap or antiseptic solution.
- Cotton.
- Sterile gauze.
- Wipes for cleaning hands.
- Painkillers (aspirin, paracetamol, ibuprofen).
- Anti diarrheal.
- Laxatives.
- Antiseptic cream.
- Antihistamines.
- Tweezers.
- Sticking plasters.
- A box with several adhesive dressings (strips).
- Sterile gauze (10 x 10 cm), wrapped separately for cleaning wounds and cover them later on.
- Round ended scissors.
- Thermometer.
- Latex gloves.
- Eye patches.
- Temporary triangle bandages.
- Thermal insulated blanket.
- Mouthpiece for administering cardiopulmonary resuscitation (optional).
- Water or 0,9 % saline solution in disposable closed containers, if there are no eyebath stations.
- Non-alcohol face wipes, if there is no water and soap.
- Plastic bags for first aid kit material that has been used or contaminated.
- According to the type of company (industry, workshop, production or manufacture of certain dangerous products, etc.), in addition to these essential elements, it is recommended to include: a stretcher, oxygen, suturing equipment, oropharyngeal tube, syringes or hypodermic needles, splints for the fracture immobilization, hemostat clamps, orthopedic collar, cold and hot compresses or hot water bag, or ice bags, knob for removing secretions, bucket for sterilizing instruments, stethoscope, nasogastric tube, medicines for strict medical control.

APPENDIX 7. WHAT TO DO IN CASE OF HAVING A WOUND

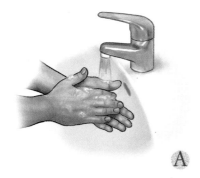

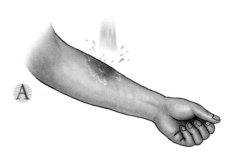

1. Wash carefully the hands with water and soap. Wash with alcohol all instruments that are going to be used: scissors, tweezers, etc.

2. Wash the wound under the tap with soap and water, softly and without rubbing in order to remove possible foreign bodies from the wound.

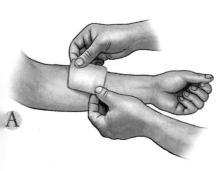

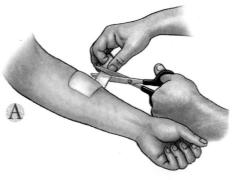

3. Use sterile gauze for cleaning the wound. It must always be done from inside to outside of the wound. Moving the gauze will be avoided the germs entrance in that wound. Sterile gauzes should not be used again.

4. It there are hairs or small pieces of skin, they will need to be cut carefully with a pair of scissors with round ended scissors.

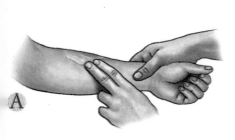

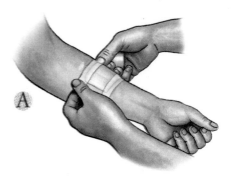

5. After that it is applied an antiseptic or iodine solution.

6. A sterile dressing will be placed on the wound in order to keep it free of germs and help the healing process. Hold the dressing with sticking plaster.

APPENDIX 8. DANGER SYMBOLS AND INDICATIONS OF DANGEROUS SUBSTANCES AND PREPARATIONS

SIGNIFICANCE AND SYMBOL	DESCRIPTION OF THE RISKS	EXAMPLES OF PRODUCTS	PREVENTIVE MEASURES
Explosive (E)	The explosion is a very fast combustion that depends on the characteristics of the product, the temperature (heating source), contact with other products (reaction), hits, frictions, etc.	Any type of sprays, even empty are potential bombs above 50°: air purifiers, hair lacquers, paintings, windshield de-icers, etc.	• Avoid the excess of heat and bumps, protect from the x rays. • Never leave these products near heat sources, lamps, radiators, etc.
Dangerous for the environment (<<N)	• Very toxic substances for the aquatic organisms. • Toxic for the fauna. • Dangerous for the ozone layer.	• Active materials of the pesticides. • Chlorofluorocarbons (CFC).	• Eliminate the product or its remains as a dangerous waste. • Avoid the contamination of the environment by doing an appropriate storage.
Toxic (T) Very Toxic (T+) Nocive (Xn)	• Harmful toxic substances and preparations that even in small amounts represent a danger for health. • If there are serious effects in the health, even for small amounts, the product is labeled with the toxic symbol. • These products penetrate the body through inhalation, ingestion or through the skin.	• Methanol, burning alcohol, stain removers. • Aerosols, waterproofing materials. • Disinfectants (creoline). • Aerosols for the vehicle paint, such as: - Stain removers, trichloroethylene, paint thinners, cleaning products. - Products for the protection and wood treatment. - Paint stripper.	• In order to avoid any contact with the skin, wear protective methods: gloves, screen, overall, etc. • Work preferably outside or in a well ventilated room. • Appropriate hygiene: wash your hands, never eat or drink when using the products. • Spray products are more dangerous (inhaling). • Keep these products out of the reach of children.
Corrosive (C)	• The corrosive substances damage seriously the life tissues and attack other materials. The reaction might be caused to the presence of water or humidity.	• Pipelines obstruction removers, descaling agents. • Caustic soda, paint strippers. • Acids, sulphuric acid (batteries).	• Keep the products in the original container (well closed containers, safety devices). • Keep these products out of the reach of children.

- Oven cleaners and toilets.
- Dishwashers products (when they are wet).

- Be careful with the place where they are left, never leave them in window sills (fall risk).
- Protect the eyes, skin, etc., against splashes. Be prudent when pouring the product or when is dusted.
- Always wear gloves and protective glasses.
- It is very important the hygiene: after using them, wash carefully face and hands.
- As a first aid, it is effective to wash with abundant water for about ten minutes.
- The aerosol corrosive products are dangerous.

Irritating (Xi)	• The repeated contact with irritating products causes inflammatory reaction of the skin and mucosa.	• Bleach. • Turpentine. • Ammonia. • Polyester filters.	• Same toxic.
Highly inflammable (F) Extremely inflammable (F+)	• (F) The highly inflammable products burn in the presence of a flame, a heat source (hot surface) or a spark. • (F+) Product that might be easily inflammable under the action of an energy source (flame, spark, etc.) even below 0°C.	• Oil, gasoline. • Burning alcohol or methanol. • Turpentine. • Mineral turpentine. • Acetone, brush cleaners, paint thinners. • Spray paint, metallic paints. • Crystal de-icer. • Contact glue, glues (neoprene). • Air purifiers.	• Store the products in a well ventilated place. • Do not use these products near a heat source, a hot surface, sparks or near a flame without protection. • Smoking is banned!. • Do not wear nylon clothes and always have a fire extinguisher located within fingertip reach when using inflammable products. • Store the inflammable products (F) well separated from the comburent products (O).
Comburent (O)	The combustion needs a combustible material, oxygen and an inflammation source: it is considerably accelerated with the presence of a comburent product (a substance rich in oxygen).	Equal inflammable products.	Equal inflammable products.

APPENDIX 9. OTHERS

ADVICES FOR SMOKING MOTHERS

- It has been scientifically that nicotine passes to the breast milk yet its levels might not be harmful for the baby. For this reason is recommended to breast-feed the baby, although the mother is a smoking mother.
- This should not be an excuse for the mother that stops smoking, which is absolutely recommended, In case the mother does not quit smoking, it is important to take into account the next advices:
  - Do not smoke inside the house, much less in the baby's room.
  - Periodically, try to reduce cigarettes consumption.
  - You should continue breast feeding, taking into account how beneficial that is the breast feeding practice.
  - Do not smoke two hours before breast feeding the baby. Despite of not being toxic, the nicotine levels for the child, far away of being beneficial, they might cause a series of harmful effects: for the stimuli effect of the nicotine, the baby of a smoking mother, possibly may have more problems for having a quiet rest and a more relaxing sleep without problems than the non smoker mother. It has also been proved that babies of smoking mothers have a higher risk of suffering the sudden death syndrome.

HOW TO PREVENT TETANUS

- The tetanus might be prevented if the vaccine has been injected, which does not protect from infection, but might protect the effects that the toxin causes.
- Anti tetanus vaccination has three initial doses, reinforcement one year later of the third dose and periodical reminder in order to keep the protection.
- The general pattern is the next: a dose at 2, 4 and 6 months of life, reinforcement at 18 months old, a reminder at 4-6 years old and a reminder every 10 years after that dose.
- In younger children than 7 years old unless it is medically contraindicated the anti diphtheria vaccination or the anti pertussis, DPT vaccine combined is used (diphtheria, tetanus, pertussis).
- In adolescents and adults the anti tetanus vaccine (T) is commonly substituted by the Td vaccination, related to the anti diphtheria in order to keep the protection against both diseases at the same time.

RECOMMENDED BIBLIOGRAPHY

NAEMT: *Apoyo Vital Prehospitalario en trauma PHTLS básico y avanzado.* 2nd ed. Comité de apoyo vital prehospitalario en trauma de la asociación Nacional de Técnica en Urgencias Médicas. México D.F., 1993.

American Heart Association: *Basic Life Support For Healthcare Providers*, 1994.

American Red Cross: *Primeros Auxilios y Seguridad para la Comunidad.* Mosby Lifeline, 1994.

Cruz Roja Mexicana: *Manual de Técnicos en Urgencias Médicas. Nivel Básico.* 3th ed, 1995.

National Safety Council et al: *Wildemess First Aid: Emergency Care for Remote Locations.* Jones & Bartlett Pub, 1997.

O'Keefe, Limmer, Grant, Murray, Bergeron: *Brady Emergency Care.* Prentice Hall, 11th ed, 1998.

Manual de Primeros Auxilios. Grijalbo-Mondadori, S.A., 1998.

Casanovas Serna E: *Manual de Primeros Auxilios.* Fraternidad, 1998.

Malagón Sisto A: *Guía de primeros auxilios.* Asociación para la Prevención de Accidentes, San Sebastián, 1999.

Martínez-Marroquín MY, García Viveros M: *Urgencias Médicas y Primeros Auxilios.* Fundación ICEPSS, 2000.

Servicios Preventivos. Formación Básica en Socorro. Cruz Roja Española, 2000.

Escuadrón SOS: *Manual para el curso básico de Técnico en Urgencias Médicas.* México D.F., 2001.

García Muñoz F: *Manual del Curso: Prevención de Riesgos Laborales.* IBERMED, 2001.

Asociación de Enfermería de Urgencias (ENA): *Enfermería de Urgencias.* Biblioteca Enfermería Profesional. 5th ed. Editorial McGraw-Hill-Interamericana, Madrid, 2001.

Conselleria de Sanidad de Galicia: *Manuel de Primeros auxilios do 061 de Galicia.* Fundación Pública Urxencias Sanitarias de Galicia 061, Santiago de Compostela, 2002.

Primeros Auxilios. Fremap, 2002.

Fernandez Ayuso D, Aparicio Santos J, Pérez Olmo JL, Serrano Moraza A (ed): *Manual de Enfermería en emergencia prehospitalaria y rescate.* Arán Ediciones, Madrid, 2002.

Álvarez C: *Manual de atención a múltiples víctimas y catástrofes.* Arán Ediciones, Madrid, 2002.

López Angón JL: *Manual de primeros auxilios: consejos para emergencias en cualquier lugar o circunstancias.* Pearson Educación, Madrid, 2003.

Cruz Roja: *Manual de primeros auxilios.* Alhambra Pearson Educación, Madrid, 2003.

Dox IG, Melloni BJ, Eisner GM: *El gran Harper Collins ilustrado.* Diccionario médico. Marbán libros, Madrid, 2005.

American Heart Association, Highlights of the 2005. AHA Guidekines for CPR and ECC. Moya MS: *Normas de actuación en Urgencias.* 3th ed. Editorial Médica Panamericana, Madrid, 2005.

Zagurski R, Bulling D, Chang R: *Programa Nebraska de primeros auxilios psicológicos.* University of Nebraska. Public Policy Center, 2005.

Cruz Roja Mexicana: *Manual seis acciones para salvar una vida.* México D.F., 2005.

Limmer D: *Emergency Care.* Earson/Pentice hall, USA, 2005.

Proehl JA: *Enfermería de Urgencias. Técnicas y procedimientos.* 3th ed. Elsevier, Madrid, 2005.

American Heart Association (AHA): *Currents in emergency cardiovascular care*, vol 16, 4 (2005-2006).

Canabal A, Navarrete P, Sánchez Izquierdo JA: *Manual de Soporte Vital Avanzado en Trauma.* 4th ed. Plan Nacional de RCP. SEMICYUC. Elsevier Doyma, 2007.

Emergency Nurses Association (ENA): *Sheehy Manual de Urgencia de Enfermería.* 6th ed. Elsevier Mosby, Madrid, 2007.

Perelló Campaner C, Gómez Salgado J (ed): *Atención enfermera en situaciones comunes en la práctica asistencial.* Enfermería Medicoquirúrgica. Colección Líneas de Especialización en Enfermería. FUDEN-Enfo Ediciones, Madrid, 2007

Vigué J, Cañas M: *Primeros auxilios*, Gorg Blanc, Barcelona 2008.

American Association of Poison Control Centers, 2008 Annual Report of the American Association o Poison Control Centers' National Poison Data System (NPDS): 26th Annual Report.

Cruz Roja: *Manual de Primeros Auxilios.* Santillana Ediciones Generales, Madrid, 2008.

http://www.terra.es/personal2/

http://www.ugr.es/~gabpca/manual.htm

http://www.americanheart.org/eccguidelines

http://www.aaaai.org/patients/gallery/foodallergy.asp.

http://www.mydocsalud.com/index.html

http://www.mayoclinic.org/first-aid

http://www.aap.org/healthtopics/earinfections.cfm.

http://www.copeson.org.mx/rbp/viaaerea.htm

http://www.aapcc.org/dnn/NPDSPoisonData/AnnualReports/tabid/125/Default.aspx.

http://www.nscisc.uab.edu/

http://www.medlineplus.gov/spanish

http://www.es.wikipedia.org/wiki/Primeros_auxilios

http://www.auxilio.com.mx/

http://www.diabetes.org/.

http://www.diabetes.org/living-with-diabetes/treatment-and-care/blood-glucose-control/hyperglyce mia.html.

http://www.ctv.es/USERS/sos/

http://www.proteccioncivilpulpi.galeonh.com/Primaux/cap1.htm

http://web.princeton.edu/sites/ehs/coldstress/coldstress.htm.

http://www.hnt.cl/p4_hospital/site/pags/2003120514745.htm

http://www.bt.cdc.gov/disasters/winter/faq.asp.

http://www.primerosauxilios.org

http://www.auxilio.com.mx

http://www.efdeportes.com/efd109/prevencion-de-riesgo-en-la-docencia-de-la-educacion-fisica.htr

http://www.epilepsyfoundation.org/about/statistics.cfm.

http://www:ssrl.juntaextremadura.net/emergencias/pdf/PrimerosAuxilios.doc

http://www.estrucplan.com.ar/producciones/entrega.asp?

http://www.sinapsis.org

http://fscip.org/facts.htm.

http://www.primeros-auxilios.idoneos.com/

http://www.saludaliaNuevo/interior/urgencias/doc/rcp/doc/rcp_pediatria.htm

http://www.medynet.com/usuarios/jraguilar/Normas%20general

http://www.semanasalud.ua.es

http://www.mayoclinic.com/health/hypothermia/DS00333/

http://www.rena.edu.ve/SegundaEtapa/ciudadania/primerosauxilios

http://mayoclinic.com./health/pink-eye/DS00258.

http://www.unirioja.es/servicios/spri/pdf/manual_primeros_auxilios.pdf
http://www.nlm.nih.gov/medlineplus/firstaid.html
http://www:bioarrayanes.cl/externos(heimlich.ppt
http://www.nlm.nih.gov/medlineplus/ency/article/000605.htm.
http://www.manualdeprimerosauxilios.com/
http://www.scif.com
http://www.iztacala.unam.mx/
http://www:fesi/.../Manual_Primeros_Auxilios.pdf
http://www.sanakit.com/descargas/primeros_auxilios_2da_parte.pdf
http://www.nlm.nih.gov/medlineplus/hypothermia.html.
http://www.rafias.com/trabajos/auxilios/auxilios1.shtml
http://www.webmd.com/first-aid/
http://www.salud.com/primeros_auxilios.asp
http://www.pe.scouts-es.net
http://www.prevenciona.com